Women's Sexual Passages

Praise for Elizabeth Davis's work

"A gold mine! It contains heart and soul and information . . . never encountered before in any form. A potent and appreciative chronicle of what it means to be a woman at home in her body . . . the more women (and men, for that matter) who read this, the more quickly our world will be healed."
—*Isabella*

"When a book on sex comes along that you think your own doctor should read, you may want to order up extra copies and pass them around at your next appointment! Enormously refreshing." —*Libido*

"An appealing mixture of medically sound fact, thorough female intuition, underhanded humor and sensitivity . . . could surprise and educate even the most sexually seasoned people." —*Moving Words/Moving Books*

"Elizabeth Davis writes vividly, succinctly, and joyously. [She] reveals a shrewd and compassionate sensitivity to women's needs. . . . "
—Sheila Kitzinger, Author of *The Experience of Childbirth, The Complete Book of Pregnancy and Birth,* and *The Place of Birth*

"Elizabeth . . . the wisdom of your work is as old as time."
—Christiane Northrup, M.D., Author of *Women's Bodies, Women's Wisdom*

I dedicate this book to my beloved daughter, Celeste, and to all young women determined to love their bodies and own their power, no matter the cost. Particularly to those in parts of the world where oppression makes this nearly impossible, I pay tribute to your small steps as acts of great vision and courage.

Ordering

Trade bookstores in the U.S. and Canada, please contact:

Publishers Group West
1700 Fourth Street, Berkeley CA 94710
Phone: (800) 788-3123   Fax: (510) 528-3444

Hunter House books are available at bulk discounts for textbook course adoptions; to qualifying community, health care, and government organizations; and for special promotions and fund-raising. For details please contact:

Special Sales Department
Hunter House Inc., PO Box 2914, Alameda CA 94501-0914
Phone: (510) 865-5282   Fax: (510) 865-4295
E-mail: ordering@hunterhouse.com

Individuals can order our books from most bookstores or by calling toll-free:

(800) 266-5592

Women's Sexual Passages

Finding Pleasure and Intimacy at Every Stage of Life

by
Elizabeth Davis

Hunter House PUBLISHERS

Library of Congress Cataloging-in-Publication Data

Davis, Elizabeth, 1950–
    Women's sexual passages : finding pleasure and intimacy at every stage of life / Elizabeth Davis; with a foreword by Germaine Greer.
        p. cm.
    Includes bibliographical references and index.
    ISBN 0-89793-292-7 (paper)
        1. Women—Sexual behavior. 2. Women—Physiology. 3. Hormones, Sex—Physiological effect. 4. Women—Health and hygiene. I. Title.
HQ29.D294 2000
306.7'082—dc21
                                              00-063147

Project Credits

Cover Design: Jinni Fontana
Book Production: ospreydesign
Copy Editor: Rosana Francescato
Proofreader: H. D. Lail
Indexer: Kathy Talley-Jones
Graphics Coordinator: Ariel Parker
Acquisitions Editor: Jeanne Brondino

Associate Editor: Alexandra Mummery
Editorial Intern: Martha Benco
Publicity Manager: Sarah Frederick
Marketing Assistant: Earlita Chenault
Customer Service Manager: Christina Sverdrup
Order Fulfillment: Joel Irons

Publisher: Kiran S. Rana

Printed and bound by Publishers Press, Salt Lake City, Utah

Manufactured in the United States of America

9 8 7 6 5 4 3 2 1   First Edition   00 01 02 03 04

Contents

Foreword

In the postwar years of the twentieth century, the power of the female stereotype was exponentially extended and intensified by mass marketing, until brassieres and high heels, nail polish and lipstick were to be found in every hovel on the globe. As the stereotype's grip tightened, resistance was born. It gathered, swelled, burst through underground channels and up into the consciousness of real women outraged and baffled by the conflicting demands made upon them. The struggle to vomit up the internalized guilt and the ingrained certainties of defect and inadequacy is not over, because male fantasy is still the deciding factor in our buying and selling. The breast-popping stereotype still dangles her four-foot legs off the car hood. The icon of the dazzling supermenial whose hands never say housework, who is always accessible to the penis and climaxes whenever her partner does (and is never without a desirous partner), and never falters on the rope bridge over the chasm of parenting, is still displayed in all our houses. But her stranglehold on female variety is gradually being loosened. Gay women have defied her way up front. Heterosexual women too, have steadily, quietly rewritten the agenda to include singleness, aging, aggression, wit, and sorrow. Character has been inscribed upon the smooth, featureless skin of the stereotype as women have demanded the right to grow up and turn into people.

The great tension at the heart of feminism has always been the pull to demand entry to the male world and claim an equal share of male characteristics, against the pressure for the right to be different but not inferior. Some feminists argued for the industrialization of motherhood and the right to carry arms in imperialist wars and to direct the bone-crushing operations of multinationals. Others wondered what real femaleness might be like, as distinct from prescribed femininity. They moved into the inscape of the gendered body, deconstructing biological femaleness not as a defect, not as a distortion of a male norm by the specific imperatives of child-bearing, but as a complex and variable norm in itself. They took to heart the biological lesson that it is not the female but the male that is the product of a defective gene.

A gifted and persistent group of women professionals set themselves the task of observing firsthand how female humans really do behave. They discovered that all kinds of received ideas about female anatomy were simply wrong, that all kinds of variation were contained within a normality far more capacious than anyone had realized before. Gradually the conviction that femaleness is a permanent disease began to lose its hold. Fathers rose from attending birthing women with a new respect for their resilience and power. Women turned away from the hospital and the clinic, looking for ways to take responsibility for their own well-being. Feminist observers put together a picture of a hitherto unknown creature, the well woman.

We still have a long way to go; the medical establishment still labors under the delusion that femaleness is a condition that demands treatment, that women's fertility is the cause of overpopulation, that machines are better at birthing than women, that wombs are something that should be extirpated, and that the menstrual cycle involves periodic insanity.

Elizabeth Davis has given women the kind of patient, loving, and respectful attention that is usually reserved for rhinos and mountain gorillas. Here is a practitioner who does not prescribe but describes, in terms that are both empowering and fascinating, the extraordinary inventiveness and variety of the human female in all her moods and phases.

Germaine Greer

Author's Note

This book springs from a fervent desire to help women understand and enjoy their sexuality, no matter what their age or situation. Gradually, we have come to understand that life is more than a simple continuum of experience; instead, it is comprised of stages quite distinct from one another, and often age-linked. These passages have been popularized by author Gail Sheehy, who helped us to understand the psychological under-pinnings of our changes by decade.

What is new here is an overview of women's sexuality not only with changes by decade, but highlighting the physiological turning points of menarche, birth, and menopause. These climactic events have been called "Blood Mysteries," because through them, women grow and become wise mysteriously, beyond reason. The scope of transformation that occurs with each of these events, and the similarities between them, have long fasci-nated me and motivated my research, and I'm pleased to have an opportu-nity to present my findings.

As the subtitle suggests, this is also a book about finding sexual pleasure. Too often, we link pleasure with guilt and cut short our enjoyment. But pleasure is important—particularly in times of overwork and mental preoc-cupation, we cannot find balance without it. In order to know pleasure, though, we must continually explore what works for us, our own unique blend of relaxation, stimulation, and release. At certain times in the life cycle, hormonal changes prompt dramatic shifts in this pleasure equation. The better we know ourselves and our bodies, the greater our chance of discovering the right mix from time to time, passage to passage.

For most women, the greatest pleasure of all comes with intimacy, in deep connection to another. Connection is the focal point of women's desire. The more we learn about neurobiology, the more we recognize this female predilection as natural, body-based. Not only in love, but in life, women want the big picture and are endlessly fascinated by how things connect and interrelate. For example, consider our usual approach to problem solving: we seek to incorporate as many factors as possible, deliberately soliciting conflicting viewpoints in order to get to the heart of the matter and distill the deep truth. This is what author Helen Fisher has termed "web thinking."[1]

This tendency may be linked to brain evolution. In primordial times, women's ability to pay attention to many things simultaneously and still stay alert was essential to rearing young in somewhat threatening circumstances. With a baby on her hip, other children clamoring for her attention, food preparation under way, and some wild beast scuffling just outside the door, a woman had to become expert at diffusing her attention, multitasking for survival. Men, on the other hand, had to stay highly focused, single-minded in hunting or defending self and kin. Women's aptitude for contextual, holistic thinking has led, over time, to high expectations of their sexual partners. In their desire for complex communication, layer upon layer, no wonder it is challenging for women today to find the depth of intimacy they long for!

Deep intimacy is understandably elusive in a society that defines sexual pleasure in terms of technique and role-playing. Most of us have had our fill of that. Nevertheless, intimacy will elude us unless we are fully intimate with ourselves. It's interesting how persistently we seek to be close to others, and yet often avoid our own deep fears in this regard. (This too may be a by-product of evolution: in hunter-gatherer days with life on the edge, who had time for self-reflection?) Yet if we long for deep intimacy and its fruits of pleasure, we must undertake the quest for self-knowledge and self-love.

How did I come to write this book? I have been a midwife, well-woman care provider, and health educator for over twenty years, and I have thus had ample opportunity to hear women's sexual stories and treat their concerns. Many of my observations and much of my data have been gleaned from my work with childbearing women. I provide not only physical care but also a large measure of education and counseling. As a mother of three, I know beyond a doubt that pregnancy, birth, and postpartum are vulnerable times for a woman, times of rapid change and adjustment. This may cause occasional estrangement between the expectant woman and her partner. I have thus been privy to the confidences and confessions of hundreds of women, recounting not only their current concerns but early, formative intimate experiences.

The need for this book became increasingly clear as I opened my practice to women of all ages, from those not yet sexually active to those well beyond menopause. Many of my clients were eager to discuss their sexual concerns, and although most wanted to talk about sex in a personal vein, many had technical questions about their bodies. Women getting off the Pill wondered about how this would affect their sex drive and were frequently concerned about changes in vaginal secretion during the monthly cycle that were entirely normal. Similarly, perimenopausal women asked about hot flashes, vaginal dryness, and dramatically fluctuating levels of desire. I found these questions to be surprisingly basic, and as I continue to hear them repeatedly, I am alarmed to think how little even the most sophisticated women know about their bodies, their hormones, their sexual makeup.

Sometimes I am faced with questions that are much more complex, involving loss of desire under circumstances of chronic stress, grief, history of abuse, or relationship upheavals. It is obvious that the bits and pieces of information most women have regarding their sexual nature are not sufficient to meet their needs. So, here is my attempt to provide an overview that links hormonal influences, the Blood Mysteries, and changes by stage of life to explore women's sexuality in a context both feminine and feminist.

My clients have not only enlightened me about women's deepest needs and desires but have helped me better understand myself. I, too, have learned to trust my own instincts, my own body-borne wisdom. This has led me to greater appreciation and trust of women in general, and to a firm belief in our capacity for self-care. Whatever problem a woman may have, I believe she herself holds the keys to its solution. It's my task to help her find relevant information and adequate support. For example, I've happily discovered that women in labor usually know better than I how to advance progress, whether through increased privacy, rest, or deep reassurance.

Beyond monitoring the physical well-being of mother and child, my role is simply to enable the laboring woman to trust her instincts and ask for what she needs. The same is true in assisting women considering elective surgical procedures, or debating whether to use allopathic medicine or some alternative therapy. I know women's strength and resourcefulness—I've witnessed it time and again. I believe in women's ability to heal themselves.

And I decry the fact that women have been severely shortchanged, handicapped by cultural mores that define them as either Madonna or Whore. Too many women have internalized these labels and now must work extremely hard to get them out of their systems. What a loss for all of us, that women's remarkable and exquisite complexity has been belittled and diminished by our culture. Yet I don't consider it premature to say that this mind-set is in decline. Although the change is nearly imperceptible in some parts of the world, the paradigm of women as the second sex is waning. Why now?

Helen Fisher, author of *The First Sex*, holds this vision of our future:

> As women continue to pour into the paid workforce in cultures around the world, they will apply their natural aptitudes in many sectors of society and dramatically influence twenty-first century business, sex, and family life. In some important parts of the economy, they will even predominate, becoming the first sex. Why? Because current trends in business, communications, education, law, medicine, government and the nonprofit sector, known as civil society, all suggest that tomorrow's world will need the female mind.[2]

Internet technology has utterly transformed our world. Communication not only has accelerated, but it has completely outgrown its old linear parameters. The Web is a web! And the business that organizes around its use must employ contextual thinking, at which women so readily excel. Thus, it is no exaggeration to say that the future depends on women's inborn abilities to incorporate diversity, take the long view, survive ambiguity, and keep loving. Power, money, and influence will be more and more available to us. Women are on their way!

* * *

The firsthand accounts in *Women's Sexual Passages* are paraphrases of comments made by my clients over the years, plus recent interview responses solicited through my women's health practice in San Francisco, California. Words cannot express the gratitude I feel toward all who have contributed to this project.

My deepest wish is that this book be useful, that it inspire women to finally set aside self-doubt and teach their partners, and their children, a true view of women's nature where the sexual aspect is no longer isolated and exploited but integrated and free. Building trust by sharing knowledge—as women have always done.

Women, Sex, and Culture

If you have ever been puzzled by your sexual mood swings, your whims, fantasies, and aversions, this book is for you! Women in civilized society have increasingly lost touch with their natural rhythms of desire, particularly in cultures dominated by male values and attitudes. Virtually our only popular reference to female sexual rhythms is a negative one, that of the undesirability of menstruating women. We will explore this taboo in depth, along with others regarding pregnancy, menopause, and sex in later years, in subsequent chapters. But first, we must define the cultural milieu that conditions our view of women's bodies and sexuality in such negative and condescending ways.

Experts on the evolution of patriarchy tell us the trouble began with the advent of an agrarian lifestyle. When we gave up our hunter-gatherer existence in favor of tending and cultivating land, ownership became an issue—particularly for men, who sought to transfer property to their male offspring. This led to claiming ownership of the mothers of their sons.

Organized religion has not helped women's struggle for equality. In the time of the Inquisition (around 1400 to 1600 A.D.), women's status in society had so deteriorated that they were considered unclean by nature, inherently sinful, and dangerous. Those women who were especially powerful—the healers, seers, herbalists, and midwives—were branded witches and were tortured, hung, or burned at the stake. *The Malleus Maleficarum*, handbook of the Inquisition, says outright, "No one does more harm to the Catholic Church than do the midwives." Here is a crucial part of history of which many of us are unaware: the holocaust of women. Estimates of the number of women who died at this time range from several hundred thousand to as many as six million. Not only did the condemned take with them a wealth of healing wisdom passed strictly by oral tradition, but their daughters and sons were forced to witness their accusation, suffering, silencing, and death. No wonder we have so much fear of women's power and embodied wisdom — it is encoded in our memories by acts of violence against our female ancestors.

And this is just European and American history. The repression of women's knowledge and power has occurred worldwide, as a result of both religious beliefs and economic factors. As capitalism forged the nuclear family, women were isolated from their kin and were forced to depend on their husbands for financial support in order to raise their young. Thus women lost their tribal ways of jointly raising children, sharing their resources, pooling their skills. Even the extended family has fallen by the wayside in many parts of the world, leaving women entirely alone to cope with their household responsibilities. If we mix in a little religious dogma — women seduce men, divert their attention from what's important, are dangerous, or are a mixed blessing at best — we have a recipe for loss of women's strength and passion.

Think about the gender myths you assimilated in childhood. Consider the overt and covert messages from the media that constantly bombard and envelop us. We've all encoded core beliefs that the feminine spells trouble through "bad girl" characters of troublemaker, slut, and fatal attractor. But the media also portray an opposite ideal of women as loving, giving, virtuous, and self-sacrificing. This is the Madonna/Whore dichotomy, set to derail any attempt at sexual holism. "Good girls" don't want sex as much as men do, but they submit for security's sake, for the sake of home and family. "Bad girls" don't care about security; they are home-wreckers and use sex, seduction, and trickery to tame and subdue their male counterparts. Thus, sex is a battleground. Men win by domination or evasiveness; women win by calculation or by being "nice."

Not much of a sexual-social legacy, is it? These suppositions are dehumanizing and demeaning to both sexes. They shape a definition of sexuality wherein feminine and masculine are mutually exclusive opposites, men and women are perpetually at odds.

Our core values regarding sex are further expressed by language. Many slang words used to describe the sex act are distinctly unpleasant to women because they portray sex as an act of male aggression toward females. These words also imply that sex equals penetration, that the penis and vagina are the primary sex organs. There are few slang words for women's sexual organs anyway, but none in common use for the clitoris. This key source of sexual pleasure and response is often left undrawn or unlabeled on anatomical sketches; girls learn the word *clitoris* much later than boys learn the word *penis*. Nancy Friday calls this tantamount to "mental clitoridectomy."[1] Natalie Angier similarly notes that in her research over a five-year period, MEDLINE scans brought up no more than sixty references to the clitoris, as compared to almost thirty times that for the penis.[2]

With regard to sexual activity, male response is the standard against which female response is evaluated and judged. When the penis is suffused with blood, we call it *erect*, but the clitoris is said to be *congested*. Even the word *vagina* comes from the Latin for sheath or scabbard, suggesting a waiting and passive receptacle for the penis. As Sheila Kitzinger, beloved authority on childbirth and women's sexuality, astutely observes, "language is either silent about women's bodies and sexuality or condemns them."[3]

Considering the above, what ever happened to the sexual revolution? What was that all about, anyway?

Contraceptive technology played a significant role in loosening sexual mores, as the Pill created new possibilities for sexual experimentation and abortion became more readily available than ever before. Never in history had consumers under the age of thirty dominated the market as they did in the 1960s. This was an era of deep idealism, bright optimism, misguided fanaticism, and genuine courage. The sexual revolution seemed promising at first, but in the end, it had very different outcomes for the sexes. Women had more opportunity to express themselves sexually, but no longer had a legitimate reason to say "no." Men, on the other hand, had the opportunity to have sex more freely than ever before without having to take responsibility. In retrospect, the primary effect was even greater pressure on women and their relationships. Yes, the sexual revolution freed women to have sex according to their passions, but those who chose not to were labeled inhibited, cold, even frigid. Cultural beliefs regarding male superiority and privilege remained unaltered, and women felt more enslaved by their sexuality than liberated to its full potential. Many learned the hard way that casual sex seldom engenders intimacy and may actually curtail any possibility of its development.

Even now, when I listen to much of what's on MTV™, I hear messages to the effect that girls are supposed to "put out" sexually, handle the wild and irresponsible behavior of their partners, and somehow cope with their own emotional responses. Doesn't sound much like liberation to me! They must also worry about sexually transmitted diseases, pregnancy, and economic dependency should they conceive. No wonder young women these days are waiting longer to become sexually active and are taking the decision to have sex much more seriously.

Underlying the polarization of the sexes is disharmony of the masculine and feminine within each of us. Regardless of gender, we all have aggressive, coolly analytical qualities traditionally considered male as well as sensitive, spontaneous qualities traditionally considered female. As we contemplate ways to harmoniously blend these aspects within ourselves, we might also question what makes men and women unique.

Groundbreaking research on this subject began with the Masters and Johnson study in 1966, which revealed for the first time women's orgasmic potential and the importance of clitoral stimulation. *Foreplay* became a household word, and although many women still feel that they don't get enough, at least they don't have to explain what it is to their partners (although they may need to give more detailed instructions). Some feel the term *foreplay* is itself problematic, as it implies that anything short of penetration is merely preliminary and therefore less significant.

But women's need for foreplay can serve as a focal point for examining a fundamental difference between the sexes. Although the vast majority of women report that foreplay is important physically, an even greater margin emphasizes the emotional benefits of feeling cared for. When foreplay occurs in a spirit of love and tenderness, it enhances physical relaxation and focus. Without this emotional component, foreplay may feel more irritating than stimulating. This brings to mind the classic dichotomy of male versus female readiness for intimacy: men need to have sex in order to feel close, while women need to feel close in order to have sex.

How much of this is cultural, how much biological? Certainly, as primary caretakers of society and its offspring, women need support, particularly in caring for the very young. In our society, the trappings of security have traditionally been provided by men. But matrilineal societies still exist where land and possessions are handed down through the woman's line, and women care collectively for one another and the children. These women are closely bonded; they are affectionate and protective of one another. This was even more the case in pre-Christian times, when conception was thought to take place by virtue of a woman's relationship to the spirit world. Because men were not considered integral to conception, women did not know or care who fathered their children and were free of the yoke of male ownership. Notably, these were peaceful cultures, with shrines and altars everywhere.[4]

It took men many thousands of years to perfect the weaponry and warfare necessary to challenge the creative power of the mothers.[5] Eventually, they exerted dominance over women as they did over one another. With the shift to land ownership, women were soon considered little more than personal property and became dependent on men for survival. Long before the Inquisition took place, women's innate capacity to heal by way of nature was usurped by men's penchant for tools, instruments, and technology.

No one really knows what female sexuality was like before cultural oppression, but we can speculate. The missionary position was probably not the first choice; perhaps women straddled their male consorts, controlling the rate and depth of penetration, generating their own foreplay. According to ancient Tantric traditions (highly reverent of women), the ideal posture of choice was entwined sitting, which allowed a slow, steady buildup of passion that could at the same time be controlled and maintained.

In any case, today we have a complex situation in which traditions of male dominance have been challenged by social upheaval. Women are no longer expected to stay at home and care for their families; they have moved fully into the workforce. Yet many have been disillusioned by the stress and strain of trying to juggle diverse roles of mother, lover, homemaker, and executive. Meanwhile, our economy has so fully adjusted to the two-income family that staying home or cutting back work hours is no longer an option for most. It would seem that women are once again trapped, doomed to overwork or to dependency on men.

Except that men, too, are eager for change. This is the new generation of fathers who have comforted crying babies in the night, changed diapers, and altered their work schedules to take care of sick children. Having done so, they've found the fast track less than appealing, and many of them want off. Public polls report that up to

70 percent of women and 40 percent of men would cut back work hours to spend more time with their families, if given the choice. This desire for increased personal time reflects our growing awareness of ebb and flow in the life cycle—we all have times of productivity and periods of exhaustion, creative spurts and phases of dormancy, and emotional ups and downs. Despite media images to the contrary, no one is perpetually active and on the go, nor should we try to be. It is no wonder that stress-related illnesses—heart disease, high blood pressure, and eating disorders—plague our society. We desperately need downtime to appreciate and enjoy life, to reconnect with our deepest passions and dreams.

How does this relate to sexuality? As the stereotypical roles of man as aggressive provider and woman as passive caretaker are outmoded, new concepts emerge of male and female needs and desires. This is true not only in the United States; even the most repressive cultures of the Middle East feel the winds of change. For example, a growing number of women activists now resist the tradition of veiling, or speak out against female circumcision. This represents a global shift in values, based on web thinking.

I recently saw a pregnancy and birth video produced in the Netherlands, and I was struck by the unusual opening sequence. This was a prolonged shot of a young couple cuddling in bed in the morning, he with his eyes closed, a smile on his face, she talking a bit and nuzzling against his cheek. Sounds like afterglow, but no, this was the tender moment when she first broke the news that she was pregnant. What struck me was that here were two equals, both of them vulnerable and strong, in touch with themselves, relaxed and communicative. To her news he responded positively, maturely, with none of that feigned idiot shock the American male often expresses upon hearing that he is going to be a father. This is undoubtedly due in large part to the fact that Holland provides both maternity and paternity leave, home nursing and housekeeping after the baby comes, and generous support—both social and financial—for the developing family.

Traditionally, European attitudes toward sex have also been much more liberal than our own, including those toward sex outside the marriage bed. For us, remnants of Puritanical mores—mind is good, body bad—lead us to view extramarital sex with more than a little guilt and confusion. Separating mind and body, denying the sensual as sacred, leads to a somewhat crude and potentially dangerous definition of sexuality. Apart from the general controversy on the subject, pornography in America must be noted for its unusual violence and brutality. When people are taught to mistrust their bodies and feelings, it's no wonder that their sexual imagery reflects that violation.

We can trace this alienation back to the Garden of Eden myth, wherein Eve made the grievous mistake of commingling with the serpent. In spiritual traditions that predate this myth, the serpent is Kundalini, the vital power of ecstasy that rises up the spine and through the top of the head when sexual energy is united with higher intelligence. My favorite T-shirt message sums it up quite nicely: "Eve Chose Consciousness." She also chose to remember her place in nature, in the circle of life. Yet to this day, most Christian religions maintain that to seek enlightenment through the body is tantamount to sin. What does this mean for women, who have no choice but to unite with their bodies in menstruation, birth, and menopause? What does this mean for all of us but neurosis, isolation, disease? To quote Susan Griffin:

> Consciousness and meaning are part of nature.... When bodily knowledge and language are separated, we ourselves experience a terrible separation that ranges all the way from grief to despair to madness.... In this way culture destroys a

woman's conscious knowledge of her own experience. Just
as she is separated from other women, from her body and
her feelings, she is, finally, a stranger to herself.[6]

Yet, against all odds, women are actively reengaging their natural
strengths and unique abilities, their propensities apart from men. They
are pulling together in circles, purging themselves of mistrust and
competitiveness. They are formulating new communication systems,
devising social structures to support them in various life phases, reani-
mating ritual celebrations from the past, or inventing new ones to suit
their present needs. The new feminism, highly personal yet imminently practical, springs from our need to unite mind and body, to
reclaim our Blood Mysteries as self-affirming and significant events
from which we derive great power.

Beyond simply acknowledging that our desire for sex depends on
our moods, which fluctuate with both biological and social influences,
lies the potential to join with our rhythms instead of working against
them, to stop denying the peaks and valleys of our existence and start
using them to enhance the quality of our lives, not only for ourselves
but for our loved ones, our culture, our world. To do so is crucial to the
survival of all living things. To my mind, woman's reunion with her
body is a metaphor for healing the planet, saving the earth.

Accordingly, we must expand our definition of sexuality to reflect
the interrelatedness of all life—the Gaia hypothesis. We are accustomed to thinking of sexuality in the most limited way, as the physical
act of intercourse alone. A more meaningful and pertinent definition
for women is so broad as to be nearly unrecognizable: Sexuality is all
that it means to be female, body and soul. This may include physical,
erotic expression, but it definitely involves the relationship of our vital
energies to other aspects of existence. Actually, the *Webster's* definition
is not far off the mark: "The sum of structural, functional and behav-

ioral peculiarities of living beings that subserve reproduction and distinguish males from females."[7]

Let us more closely examine these "behavioral peculiarities" that distinguish women from men. To what extent might these be biologically based? The data show that numerous gender-specific characteristics reveal themselves in early infancy, long before acculturation takes place. For example, most baby boys demonstrate a much stronger attraction toward tangible objects than do girls, who are more interested in the human face, in communication. Men see better in bright light and at a distance, but women literally see the big picture: we have wider peripheral vision due to extra rods and cones at the back of the retina. And when it comes to tactile sensitivity, even the least sensitive woman is more sensitive than the most sensitive man (this is one area in which test scores of each sex don't even overlap).[8]

At the root of these gender-specific traits are differences in brain structure and function that further distinguish the sexes. This is new information for the general public but old news to the neuroscientists. For many years, funding was unavailable for research in this area, so pervasive was the belief that cultural influences were the last word in character development. And there was also legitimate concern on the part of female researchers that the data might be used to argue male superiority. But the ongoing philosophical debate among leading female thinkers underscores the need for this information.

In 1990, Susan Faludi made waves with her book *Backlash: The Undeclared War Against American Women,* by documenting how commonly data have been used to undermine women's gains and accomplishments. To some extent, she perpetuated a feminism that took its aim at men, one that called for sweeping changes in male values and behavior. Then Camille Paglia, author of *Sexual Personae,* declared this sort of feminism self-indulgent and simplistic, fraught with unrealistic expectations of what men must do in order for women to find true equality. "Women will never know who they are until they let men be men," she stated, at the same time deriding feminists as self-pitying whiners who just needed to get on with their lives.[9] With this polarization, the promise of female autonomy remained elusive, until neurobiological research was brought to public awareness by such authors as Christiane Northrup, Helen Fisher, and Natalie Angier. These women share a common passion to define woman on her own terms, rather than in relationship to the male of the species. In their work, they place emphasis on what is right with women, rather than pointing the finger at men, thus diffusing some of feminism's excesses and mistaken assumptions. They agree that patriarchy is a problem, but men are not the target.

To return to the research on brain structure, we now know that the fetus produces hormones at about six weeks' gestation that differentiate the sex organs and affect brain development. In 50 percent of females, the prefrontal cortex becomes thicker than it does in males. The cortex contains control centers that govern behavior; in the male, functions are highly specialized—"lateralized"—according to hemisphere, but in the female, functions are diffused, replicated on both left and right sides of the brain. An outstanding example is that of the emotional centers, which in women are found in both hemispheres but in men are located on the right side only. Add to this the fact that men have verbal centers only in the left hemisphere, and we see a biological basis for the difficulty men tend to have in expressing their feelings.[10]

Most men show a decided preference for the left side of the brain— associated with linear thinking—whereas women regularly access both hemispheres. Since the right side of the brain has more connections with the body than does the left, women have more access to the body-based wisdom when thinking and speaking than do men.[11]

This ability of women to switch easily from one side of the brain to the other results from an enlargement of the parts of the brain that connect the two hemispheres—the corpus callosum and the anterior commissure.[12] This may explain women's ability to handle several tasks simultaneously, while men prefer to focus on one thing at a time. Women's attention is generally more diffused, multifaceted, than is men's. Thus, our approach to problem solving is to encircle, to consider a problem from a variety of angles before moving to the center for a solution. Men tend to break things down and categorize as they solve problems, adding up factors methodically, bricklayer-style. This is why, when the sexes try to solve problems together, men are at a loss to understand why women bring in so many seemingly unrelated factors and can't get to the point, while women wonder why men must be so controlling and tight-lipped—what's wrong with talking things through? Women by nature tend to expand, while men contract.

We can readily extrapolate these tendencies to differences in sexual needs. In his groundbreaking book *Men, Women and Relationships*, author John Gray suggests that a basic misunderstanding of key differences between the sexes is at the root of most sexual unhappiness and dysfunction. What does a woman need from a lover? Assistance in focusing! Especially after a busy day, she needs help in bringing her diffused and expanded awareness back to focus on herself, her body. It has been shown that women need an average of eighteen minutes of stimulation to reach orgasm, whereas men need only two or three.[13] Women need cuddling, they need to be touched in a nonsexual way at first, erogenous zones aside.

Gray further observes that the delicious, total-body pleasure felt by women with this warm-up is usually experienced by men only after they climax, because men tend to focus and contract their sexual tension until they ejaculate. Both sexes can help each other by recognizing and balancing their differences; he, by taking the time to help his partner relax, she, by making the wait enjoyable for him or by being up for an occasional "quickie."

But apart from our relationships with men, we women have our own inherent mechanisms for growth and exploration: our biological rhythms. The monthly cycle moves us through an exquisite sequence of moods and passions; each time around, we experience the spectrum. Menstruation is the *petite morte*, the end of one cycle and the beginning of another. This is our time to reflect on lingering disappointments and frustrations in our lives, and to have another go at their resolution. Menstruation also links us to the rhythms of the moon, which profoundly influence our earthly existence. Later, when we no longer have need of the monthly cycle because we've learned its lessons through and through, we cease menstruating and retain our "wise blood" for the benefit of society. These biological imperatives give our lives meaning; they are vehicles for vision, for transformation.

Yet all of this may be negatively affected by our culture's determination to keep us in a caretaking role. Women do have some biological predilection to nurture, but this has been grossly exploited by society. Remember that in patriarchal systems such as ours, women are subordinate and are held responsible to men before themselves. Thus, scientific evidence of hormonal prompts for maternal instinct and behavior has been turned against women, used as a gauge of femininity, despite the fact that there is no indication that these nurturing behaviors extend in any significant degree to the care of grown men, let alone those outside the immediate family.

Nevertheless, women have for generations been made to live their lives through others. Their worth has been contingent on how well they foster male superiors: "Behind every good man, there's a good woman." If there are problems in the family, guilt and blame invariably fall on the woman. She is responsible for making it work: discerning problems, implementing solutions, and blending everything in perfect harmony. Predictably, this task consumes whatever time she might otherwise find for herself. And how is she expected to

respond to all this? She is to be self-sacrificing, stoic, faithful, complacent to life's "realities," yet willing and able to fight fiercely for her kin.
Though ludicrous to many of us today, the social construct persists.

If we nurture others to the exclusion of ourselves, we inevitably
attempt to live out our dreams and desires through them as well. As
the contemporary saying reminds us, "Women marry hoping to
change their partners; men marry hoping their partners will never
change." We must, once and for all, see this for what it is: a recipe for
loss and disappointment. Only by establishing our own needs and
goals as priorities can we hope to find fulfillment in life. Although we
may nurture and care for others to some extent, let this be by choice
rather than by obligation.

In light of all this, it is hardly surprising that although women are
better educated and more sophisticated now than at any time in recent
history, we remain puzzled by and thus at the mercy of our biological
rhythms, unable to incorporate them into our lives. This is largely
because these rhythms engender an ebb-and-flow approach to living
distinctly at odds with the male "ladder of success" model. But it seems
the time has come for us to share with our partners and society a truer
definition of what it means to be a woman. These are the things
women know: that everything comes around, that reflection is
germane to creative action, and that the passage of time alone can be
a key factor in change. We have learned these things organically
through the monthly cycle, in gestating our young, in weathering the
stages of marriage and child rearing, in transforming through
menopause. As society cries out for balance, for solutions to major
crises in health care, education, and our environment, women's
wisdom is once again coming to the fore. Women are speaking out,
acting up, "walking their talk," and making the difference.

Sexual
Awakening

When was your first experience of sexual awakening? Not necessarily your first sexual interaction, but your own experience of coming alive to your sexual nature?

This may be a bit hard to pin down, because sexuality is with us from birth. Even as infants, we are saturated with the "love hormone" oxytocin when breast-feeding. One woman compared her first orgasm to the feeling of ecstasy and physical release she experienced when walking through puddles as a child. Some of us remember the first time we touched ourselves sexually, or perhaps were touched by another in a spirit of play and exploration.

The first time I can ever recall having a feeling of what society calls arousal is when I was about four years old. I would use the palm of my hand and roll it up into a fist and sit on it and rub back and forth until I had an orgasm. Sometimes I would use a towel, a blanket, or anything that was around me. When I was five years old, my twelve-year-old brother caught me "wiggling" (that's what he called it) and said he was going to tell my mom and that I was going to be in big trouble. I was ashamed and embarrassed that he caught me, and I really didn't want my mother to know what I had been doing. A few days later my mom and I were on a walk and she asked me if I knew what the terms *wiggling* or *humping* meant. Of course, I denied everything.

I was in the fifth grade now and still humping and wiggling. I was constantly aroused, it seemed. Whatever I was doing, I knew I had this little secret that could make me feel so good inside, and I always wanted to use it. It never mattered when those feelings came on. If I was in school, I would get a hall pass to go to the bathroom and would wait

until no one was in there, then I would get on the floor and
sit on my hands until I felt great.

Masturbation is with us from a very early age. Books on child care
typically reassure parents not to worry if their one-year-old son plays
frequently with his penis, or if their baby daughter often has her hand
between her legs. But if the hormones associated with sexual maturation and the sex drive are not present to a significant degree, why does
this happen? Again, the answer is oxytocin. This hormone is released
not only with direct genital contact, but at the mere thought of physical pleasure. Oxytocin has been called the "bonding hormone,"
because it engenders feelings of desire, tenderness, affection, and intimacy.

Billy Adams touched me. I'll never forget it! I was very
young, maybe seven years old. We locked ourselves in the
bathroom and played doctor. He examined me. It's all sort
of a blur in my memory except the moment when he
touched me. I had never felt anything before that brought
me so into the present and opened me up to my place in
nature all in the same instant. Unfortunately, that moment
was cut short. We were discovered just as he was touching
me, and he was sent home. We were not allowed to play
together anymore. Too bad. I could have learned a lot about
myself and my body right then in a very sweet and innocent
way.

From then on, I kept feelings of where I fit in nature very
private, thinking they were wrong and bad. I always thought
there was something wrong with me for thinking about my
place in nature and my body as just a part of it, the same as
a dog or raccoon.

In spite of the naturalness of our promptings, many of us are made to feel guilty and ashamed by our first sexual impulses. This is particularly true of girls, whose parents feel they must do whatever possible to keep them from getting interested in sex too soon, lest unplanned pregnancy occur. Nevertheless, curiosity about sex happens when it will, often at a much earlier age than sex-ed programs in the schools reflect.

> My sexuality was shaped greatly by the era I grew up in. My mother was a flower child, a hippie; the sexual revolution was still in full effect in her life. I was raised in a communal situation for the first six years of my life, and I think I must have witnessed some sexual affection between my parents or their friends—it would have been pretty difficult not to, living and traveling in a school bus together up the West Coast! I have hazy memories of hearing my mom make noises with my dad that I now know to be sex/pleasure sounds. I was definitely curious as to what they were doing, and I can remember calling out and asking them one particular night.

> Later on, I remember being in the third or fourth grade, sneaking into the living room to watch TV in the middle of the night, turning it down so low I had to strain to hear the dialogue. We had cable, and I found *Lady Chatterly's Lover* on Showtime. My whole body knew this was a movie I should not be watching, but I had to see it through. That was the first time I had ever really seen sex. The movie sent feelings through my body that I had no clue what to do with. This was what everyone did in their bedroom?

And another account:

My sexuality was completely formed by society, TV, magazines, and older friends. Even when I did not know what sex was, I knew it had to do with males and females being close and comfortable with each other. When I think back to what I first thought about sex, I thought it had nothing to do with the woman's pleasure; it was purely to satisfy the man, and women just had to do it in order to be loved.

After many questions and much research, I discovered it had something to do with the vagina and the penis. Even at the age of six or seven I was able to put two and two together and figure out that if a man could do it, I most definitely could do it by myself. So one night I explored. I remember feeling funny, but I kept telling myself, "It's your body, you shouldn't feel funny touching it." That was the night I discovered my very own sexuality.

From these accounts, we can surmise that girls become sexually awakened at quite a young age, and that most would appreciate clear and accurate information on the subject much sooner than we tend to provide it. It is also poignantly evident that for us to impart a sense of guilt or shame to a girl regarding her sexual behavior can have a devastating effect on her self-esteem. She can stop neither her sexual drives nor her sexual curiosity, but if she learns to associate these impulses with wrongdoing, her opinion of herself will inevitably decline. Recall from Chapter 1 women's contextual, relational tendencies in learning, in life—much more so than boys, girls take to heart the feelings and opinions of others.

This brings to mind the wonderful work of Carol Gilligan, and her book *In A Different Voice*. In her research, Gilligan found that girls reach a critical point around the age of nine or ten when they begin to doubt their natural instincts and abilities. As a result, they lose their "voice"—that is, their ability to speak up for themselves and maintain their own opinions. Interestingly enough, this is not as contemporary a phenomenon as we might think, but dates back to the early 1900s.[1]

Why is this so? Remember that girls develop very differently than boys. Even at birth, the brains of each differ in structure and function. In boys, the left hemisphere of the cortex tends to develop much more rapidly than in girls, who have relatively equal development in both hemispheres. In other words, girls have an inherent balance of the nonlinear, intuitive aspects of the right hemisphere and the linear, logical aspects of the left hemisphere.[2] When given aptitude tests on ethical decision-making, girls tend to score lower than boys precisely because they see the big picture, bringing in so many variables that their answers are considered too vague to score. Again, this contextual, relational way of thinking comes naturally to girls, but when they realize it is not valued by our society, they either quiet down or just give up.[3]

As we try to support our daughters and help them mature, it is crucial that we teach them to resist this culturally based oppression, lest it turn into suppression of their own instinctive wisdom. How can we do this? Notice that the age at which girls tend to lose their voices dovetails with the average age of menarche (the first menstruation). This is more than a coincidence. As is true of all the Blood Mysteries, the period leading up to the main event is charged with emotion, chaos, uncertainty; in approaching menarche, girls typically become uppity and outspoken. This is a grand opportunity for us to bear witness and stand by supportively, encouraging their candor and forthrightness. Many cultures formalize this major life transition with ceremony and celebration. And in most such ceremonies, women of all ages welcome the young woman into the community at large. For ideas on how to develop a Menarche Rite, see the box on page 34.

More than any time in recent history, young women are interested in hearing stories from their elders. Storytelling is oral tradition, and as such bears different meaning from what we read in books. The story-teller is just as much a part of the story as the setting and events. When experienced women tell their young cohorts stories of their own Blood Mysteries, their menarche, birth, and menopause experiences, they help them to see the continuity of these events reflected in who they are, what they have become.

Once a girl has reached the age of ten, she becomes increasingly socially identified and needs more than her mother's counsel. Most girls get their information from TV, the Internet, magazines, movies, and so on. The stories and advice of other female relatives or wise friends can help to counterbalance negative imprints.

Returning to menarche for a moment: What is happening to a girl at the physical level? She experiences surges of estrogen, progesterone, and testosterone for many months before levels stabilize sufficiently to initiate menstruation. To experience menarche she must also have enough body fat, at least 17 percent of her total body weight (this is why anorexic, extremely thin, or highly athletic young women often do not menstruate, a condition known as amenorrhea). For sustained menstruation and regular cycles, a young woman needs about 22 percent body fat. Her first cycles may be anovulatory (meaning that no egg is released), but gradually her body will catch on and her cycle will be established.

The average age of menstruation is creeping downward; it is not uncommon for girls today to experience menarche at age ten. Just a few decades ago, the average was age twelve. What is happening here? It appears that a potent combination of chemical estrogens in our envi-ronment and growth-stimulating hormones in dairy products may be causing menarche to occur earlier and earlier (see Chapter 3 for more details). Our girls are literally being forced to grow up before they are emotionally ready. All the more reason for treating menarche as a rite of passage. Consider the following account:

I remember wanting to get my period because then I'd be a woman and I felt like, *wow*. I used to go to these meetings with my mom and the older women would talk about it, it was such a common thing that was always talked about. PMS, you know—they'd kid around about it. When my mom's friends bled at the same time, it was like this really bonding thing between them, and I always wanted to be a part of that. And then I got my period—I woke up and I was so excited! I had just started seventh grade, and I felt so much older and wiser.

The Menarche Rite was my mom's idea. She had read about it and brought the idea home to me. At first I didn't want to do it because it was my own private thing, but then I thought it might be fun. My mom and I talked about it and I read lots of books about it, and then we started to plan the ritual. I was having so much fun with it. I was really excited about this high-mark rite where I could become a woman, and all my closest friends and all the women that had always been closest to me all my life would be there.

We planned it out on note cards. Everybody had different things they would do. We made an altar with family photo-graphs of all the women before me. My mother and I brought flowers. We made another little altar in the middle of the table with tampons and pads all over it and candles— it was so beautiful. I had a beautiful silk dress my mother had gotten for me. I was totally in a daze, I just loved it! It was *my* ritual! I felt grown up, part of the circle of women.

Now I look at my bleeding as a natural thing and not at all a pain in the ass. Lots of my girlfriends groan and say, "Oh, God, I've got my period," like it's a bad thing. I look at it as such a beautiful thing that millions of women have gone through, and the ritual made me feel that way. I have my menarche box at home with all my stuff in it—I'm really thankful for that.[4]

I strongly believe that a young woman's experience of menarche affects the quality of her first sexual encounter. If her menarche is honored, especially by the elders of her community in a way that also has meaning to her, she is apt to respect her body and herself too much to casually surrender her virginity. Unfortunately, a high percentage of young women have unhappy first experiences.

I really loved this guy, and had certainly had opportunities before to be sexual with others, but for me, he was the one. I was just fifteen, and he was nineteen, already in college. We went off to a friend's beach house, and he fixed me a drink (my first one) and we took a shower together. One thing led to another, and the moment came.

Even though it didn't hurt that much, I guess because I'd already masturbated and had things inside me, I didn't feel much of anything. He actually accused me of not being a virgin, which made me feel awful. He didn't call me for two weeks, and then he was distant. Later, through a friend, I found out he was getting married to someone else. I carried the torch for a while . . . then gave it up. It was two years before I had sex with anyone else.

Another account:

Starting when I was eight years old, my brothers and I were sent to our grandmother's house for several summers because our mom was sick and couldn't deal with three little kids at the time. We slept in the back room after spending all day at the beach. My oldest brother, who was twelve, would put his hand or his mouth under the covers at night and play with me. I liked the feeling, but felt very naughty for liking and wanting it. Because of this conflict, I felt paralyzed and didn't do anything, I just lay there and let him do want he wanted to me. That feeling of paralysis, not being able to say what I want and don't want, left me feeling powerless.

My brother's desires for me escalated as he grew into his teens. I began to feel that the only way to be liked by a man was to give him whatever he wanted of my body.

This account is not only disturbing but crosses the line into incest. Yet many young women report first sexual encounters with older brothers. Where are their mothers, why can't they tell them, and why aren't their mothers aware?

And another, equally distressing:

When I was seventeen I had been dating a boy for three months, and he wanted to know how much longer I was going to hold out before giving it to him. I wasn't sure I wanted to take my pants off, and why should I? I knew I could make myself feel great just by kissing and rubbing back and forth on his penis through my clothes. He said that caused him great pain and that if I thought that felt great, just wait until the real thing. I was scared. I did love him and I didn't want him to leave just 'cause I wouldn't take my pants off.

One week later I gave it up to him, and it was nothing like the great secret I had of making myself feel good. I was in a lot of pain, there was bleeding, there were tears, and there was no orgasm. I was thoroughly disappointed with him, with society and with myself for giving up something that was so special to me for ninety seconds of sheer terror.

Why are these initial experiences so often unsatisfying? If a woman is partnered with a young man, he will often rush to intercourse without adequate foreplay. As Theresa Crenshaw points out in her book *The Alchemy of Lust*, sexual exploration just shy of intercourse invariably involves lots and lots of kissing, holding, petting, and fondling, which serves to dramatically increase oxytocin levels in both partners. When this prolonged period of foreplay is either replaced by intercourse or cut short, women in particular miss the closeness and bonding engendered by high levels of oxytocin.[5]

They may also miss orgasm altogether. According to a study recently conducted at the University of Chicago involving three thousand participants aged eighteen to thirty-nine, 25 percent of women were unable to achieve orgasm during intercourse.

Psychologist Alfred Ellis, author of the book *Restoring Innocence*, observes that first sexual experiences have tremendous power to imprint us either for good or ill. In this case, imprinting refers to a process of deeply internalizing the attitudes and beliefs of an intimate partner under mutual circumstances of great stress or extreme excitement. Ellis believes that first-lover imprints can influence sexual behavior and the capacity for sexual enjoyment for many years to come.

Here is a young woman's story that demonstrates how positive feelings about her body and herself contributed to a positive first experience. Although not specifically mentioned, it seems clear that an open and loving relationship with her mother played a significant part in her ability to wait to have sex until she was truly ready:

> I had my first kiss at age fourteen with my boyfriend. I felt a whole new arousal in making out with him and had my first orgasm fully clothed, rubbing our bodies together. We explored each other's bodies, went skinny-dipping in his pool, and I had my first intense orgasm during oral sex when we snuck away during a camping trip with my family. This was the first time I remember feeling out of control, an out-of-body erotic feeling. Once I started to experience orgasms, I realized I could do it by myself. I found my mother's vibrator and used it every so often, or the lid from my teen perfume, Love's Baby Soft.

> About masturbation, my mother had a talk with me once and I remember her saying that it was okay to do, it was natural. At some point, I got influenced by other sources and I would sometimes feel guilty doing it so often. This wore off as I grew older and formed my own beliefs.

> I began to feel more sexy. I loved dancing nude in front of the mirror, I loved the way my body looked and the way the curves felt. I dated a lot and experimented with guys as much as one can and without having intercourse. During my junior year, I started dating my old boyfriend again. After six months, I decided that even if he wasn't "the one," I did love him, and I wouldn't regret losing my virginity to him. We discussed birth control, and I talked to my mother about it and decided on a diaphragm. I was fitted for one, and we set a date. A romantic weekend at his parent's cabin, with gifts and champagne, and he was so gentle that I had an orgasm that first time.

This young woman, aged nineteen, also had a positive first experience and had this to say to other young women hoping to have the same:

> I think sex is looked on much too lightly in this society, I believe this to be one of the most detrimental outcomes of our society's way of expressing itself in the twenty-first century. Sex is a sacred act that not only invades a woman's body but makes it very possible that she could be carrying a baby in her belly for the next nine months, labor that baby into the world, and be a mommy for the rest of her life. In my opinion, we should not have any mommies who do not want to be, or are not ready to be, mommies.
>
> As I casually flip through the channels on TV, I am appalled at what I see. I don't think there is one show on TV these days that portrays that it is not only okay, it is a woman's right not to sleep with a man on the first date. Sex should be portrayed not only as a woman's right, but as a man's privilege to enter her most sacred temple, her body. On TV, if a woman does decide to open her sacred body to a man she has barely known for two hours, she is not expected to gain much from this experience: she *of course* will not have an orgasm, but he *of course* will completely get off.
>
> My heart goes out to all the young girls growing up in our society today, molding their sexuality to what they see on TV, and comparing themselves to these unempowered women, or dolls, I should say, in the magazines. What a hard struggle it will be for them to find their true identity and discover that they're only as unique and beautiful as they make themselves out to be. That their sexuality is their own, and their body, a temple to be entered only by the most sacred individual in their eyes.

How can we reinstill a sense of the sacred into sexuality? I think one of the best ways is to teach young women more about the power and beauty of their bodies at a basic physical level. Old imagery of the female body as a passive vessel for male pleasure must be replaced with new scientific findings that show quite the opposite to be true.

For example, standard explanations of the process of conception purport that the egg is passive, almost stupid, indiscriminately waiting to be penetrated by whatever sperm comes along. But more recent observation of the process by fiber optics shows the egg to be quite selective, chemically rejecting a considerable number of sperm until finally permitting one to come inside:

> That thick, extracellular coat [of the egg] is the famed zona pellucida—the translucent zone—the closest thing a mammalian egg has to a shell. The zona pellucida is a thick matrix of sugar and protein that is as cunning as a magnetic field. It invites sperm to explore its contours, but then repels what doesn't suit it. It decides who is friend and who is alien.[6]

The cervix also plays a role in conception only recently revealed by fiber optics. Quite the opposite of the immobile, passive organ we once envisioned it to be, it actually dips up and down as the uterus contracts during orgasm. In this, there is a link to a woman's chance of conceiving. If her partner ejaculates and she orgasms soon after, her cervix will dip repeatedly into seminal fluid pooled at the end of her vagina, drawing it up inside her. Timing is everything—and the cervix actively participates.[7] And apparently, there are more than emotional factors involved when a woman whose partner has already climaxed decides to "go for it" herself.

Young women also need a deeper understanding of the role of the clitoris in pleasure and orgasm. Another common misconception is that, with stimulation, the clitoris gets erect just like the penis. But recent studies show that the clitoris lacks a venous plexus, which in men prevents blood from flowing out of the aroused penis. In women, blood flow in and out of the aroused clitoris is flexible and fairly continuous, which makes it more adaptable to varying degrees of stimulation, able to distend and relax quickly. This accounts for women's marvelous ability to have multiple orgasms during a single sexual encounter.[8]

Last but not least, women need a better understanding of the vagina: how it is strong, how it is vulnerable. As Natalie Angier brightly declares, "The vagina is its own ecosystem, a land of unsung symbiosis and tart vigor."[9] Women everywhere are still taught that the vagina is dirty, but it is actually quite clean—cleaner than the mouth. Yes, the vagina is full of bacteria, but they are healthy lactobacilli organisms (like those found in yogurt) that literally eat back offending types. Normal vaginal discharge is just that—normal. It is composed of the same ingredients as blood serum (what is left in blood when the red cells are separated out).

What causes vaginal infection? Ironically, a major cause is douching. This practice, which is supposed to leave us feeling "clean and fresh," actually puts us at risk by washing away those friendly lactobacilli we need for vaginal health. Another cause of vaginal infection can be sex itself, especially for the heterosexual woman who has not been active for a while or is with a new partner. Vaginal pH is normally quite acidic, around 3.8 to 4.5; seminal fluid is alkaline, with a pH around 8. Sudden exposure to highly alkaline seminal fluid may cause an overgrowth of yeast organisms normally present in the vagina in limited amounts. With a new (male) partner, there may also be an immunological reaction to alien sperm, if only at first.

Returning to the theme of masturbation, it is vitally important that every young woman realize the freedom and pleasure to be had in this harmless practice. As a society, we don't exactly frown on masturbation, but we certainly don't condone it. Yet it is a clear alternative for women not yet ready to be sexually active, or for those taking a sexual time-out.

My sexual coming of age was sort of a "group effort." My housemate's boyfriend bought her the book *Sex for One*, by Betty Dodson, and it soon made its way around the house. We were all in our late teens or early twenties and had experimented with masturbation, but Betty opened our eyes to a whole new sexual arena: the *vibrator*.

I remember the first night I used it. Taking the advice of good ol' Betty, I took a bath to relax, because I knew I had an audience in the other room waiting for a rave review. Even though I had masturbated before, I had never had an orgasm, and I really didn't expect to have one right away. Several months later, I actually did. I was blown away, to say the least. It made me so happy to know that I didn't have to depend on another person for sexual satisfaction. Since I was the only one of my friends that was still a virgin, I was beginning to think my sex life would never get off the ground. Using the vibrator totally changed all that. I especially liked knowing that in the blink of an eye I could run up to my room and get myself off. No one could stop me, and I didn't need anyone to help me either. My sexuality was *mine* now. I felt like I held a great power that women have not tapped into, for whatever reason.

Knowing that my sexuality is *mine*, I view sex a bit differently. I still feel it is something to be held sacred between those involved. But now, knowing the power I feel in my own sexuality, I want to share it with different people. I feel more comfortable being intimate with others, maybe because I don't play mind games with myself as I used to, or maybe because I am so much more mature than I used to be.

Self-discovery, self-affirmation, and self-respect are the cornerstones of a young woman's sexual maturation. Even if she has a rocky start with menarche or her first love is a disappointment, she can still find her way, especially with the help of other women. Here is a story of one woman's transformation:

> The stories I heard in quiet corners with hushed voices were horror stories about how each woman in our family was handling the "curse." It was clear from the beginning that having your period was not anything to be happy about. I was given detailed instructions on how to deal with this "menace," for if I did not, I would suffer greatly like those before me. Cramps, bloating, huge blood loss, headaches, fainting spells—the list went on and on.
>
> For the next seven years I popped pills, made sure every tampon was deodorized, and kept constant vigilance on my calendar lest some fun activity present itself when I was expecting to bleed. Needless to say, this behavior of self-abhorrence left its mark on my relationships. I completely denied my feminine self and wanted to be one of the guys. I was built athletically and was highly competitive, and I considered most women to be weak, "frilly," and only concerned with "simple" things.
>
> What I didn't understand until much later was that because I had rejected my biology and my femininity, my relationships with men would be little more than a reflection of my self-loathing. If I couldn't enjoy my body as a woman, I couldn't enjoy sex—although I thought I was at

the time. Basically, though, I was there to please. Not even thinking that I had desires. Men were the ones who needed sex; I just played along.

After several years of falling and getting back up again, I became aware of the deep-seated hatred I had for women. I especially disliked women who enjoyed the arts of cooking, sewing, baking, and child rearing. Women who were vulnerable, loving, and open to truly experience life would push my buttons and make me really uncomfortable. Then, after I had my son, I came to realize that deep down in me was that woman—I love to cook, bake, be with my son, love deeply, garden, sculpt, and paint. My cycle took on a whole new meaning for me. I started wearing natural cotton menstrual pads instead of tampons, saving my blood in a menstrual bowl and giving it back to the earth. I'd take the entire first day of my flow and do whatever felt right, holding it as a sacred time in my life. I changed my viewpoint and also my words—words have power. I now practice the art of fertility awareness. I touch and smell my body daily; it is a temple to me now.

As I was starting these practices, I noticed a shift in my perception of other women. No longer would I walk down the street and try to make eye contact with a man who was walking with another women. Instead, I made eye contact with her. I grew to love women, because I was growing to love myself.

In the next chapter, we will learn more about how women are reclaiming the menstrual cycle, including the sexual peaks it engenders.

The Menarche Rite

Women have definite physiologic milestones that herald major life transitions. There was a time when these transitions were held holy and served to connect us with the rhythms and cycles of the seasons and the moon. The first of these milestones is the Menarche Initiation Rite, held at the time of a young woman's first menses to honor her crossing from girlhood to womanhood.

In the past, it was customary to mark this major change in a woman's life with a special observance or celebration. Anticipation of this honoring helped the girl greet her first bleeding with joy and triumph; it was the most essential of all initiation rites.

In nonindustrial societies, seclusion is a nearly universal component of the menarche rite, not out of fear but in reverence for the sacred power of menstrual blood. In some indigenous cultures, girls are isolated for several years. Young Dyak women of southeast Asia spend a year in a white cabin, wearing white clothes and eating white foods only (thought to ensure good health.)[10] While alone, they contemplate their physical transformation to womanhood and consider what society expects of them. Elder women visit periodically to teach the art and craft of womanhood, including the responsibilities of sexuality and child rearing. This has enormous impact on their personal growth.

One of the most beautiful examples of menarche initiation is the Apache rite of "Changing Woman." In this solemn ceremony, the pubescent girl becomes the primordial Apache mother, "White Painted Woman." She reenacts the story of Changing Woman who, impregnated by the sun, gave birth to the Apache people. On the first day, she is sprinkled with yellow cattail pollen to symbolize fertility, and is taught by wise-women of the "fire-within," her sacred sexuality. The ceremony lasts for four days, in honor of the Four Directions. On the final night, the young woman must dance from sunset to sunrise for the well-being of her people. At dawn, this song is sung to her:

> "Now you are entering the world.
> You will become an adult with responsibilities…
> Walk with honor and dignity.
> Be strong!
> For you are the mother of our people…
> For you will become the mother of a nation."[11]

Although a four-day ritual may seem excessive in the context of our busy lifestyles, its purpose of enabling young women to experience heightened awareness of their new status and power is highly relevant. Menarche rites of today can range from formal ceremony to a simple gathering of special women friends and relatives for a wonderful meal together. The main idea is to distinguish this milestone event from everyday life. Women across the country are busy recreating or inventing these ceremonies for their daughters. But it is crucial that young women themselves participate in the design and content of their celebrations, choosing what is comfortable for them. Here are some suggestions for a memorable event.

The place where the celebration will be held can be decorated with candles and flowers of red and white, red symbolizing blood and life force, white representing innocence, strength, and reproductive health. The young woman may wish to sit at the place of honor, the head of the table perhaps, with her chair decorated like a throne. The centerpiece might be red roses, one for each year she has lived. She may also want to wear a crown of flowers, signifying her flowering womanhood.

To begin, the group can acknowledge and invoke the young woman's ancestors, all the women in her family line who have crossed this threshold before. This affirms her place in the community of women, her procreative potential, and the natural beauty of her menarche experience.

The body of the rite involves sharing information on menstruation through storytelling and first-person accounts. Each woman present is given the opportunity to describe her menarche experience. Not all of these stories will be joyous; older women may become very emotional if they recall feeling ashamed of their first blood. Yet this creates even stronger intent within the circle to honor the young woman currently in the midst of this Blood Mystery.

An ancient form of honoring menarche is the Clay Rite, similar to the Apache use of cattail pollen. This is only appropriate if the young woman feels comfortable enough to be nude in the presence of her friends. Those who have not yet started bleeding cover her with wet, red clay, to symbolize her connection to the earth. This can be fun—a playful, messy act of saying farewell to childhood.

If they are in a rural setting, the group may wish to construct a sweat lodge for the young woman, where she may spend a certain amount of time in seclusion. As an alternative, she might spend a night alone in a tent or cabin with her friends close by, singing or drumming to give her courage. Or she might simply go off by herself for a time to a place of total privacy.

After a while, several "wise women" or a special relative come to her with instructions regarding her fertility and responsibilities in the next stage of life. When they are finished, she returns to the larger group. Her friends may wish to form a birth arch at this point, lining up and passing the young woman through their legs until she finally comes to her mother, who brings her out and into her embrace. As with actual birth, there is a moment in this act where time seems suspended—the power of this ritual is tangible.

The "newborn" woman may then be washed clean of remaining mud by those of her friends who have already begun bleeding, welcoming her into the adult community of women. She should then be dressed in new, beautiful clothing she can treasure for years to come, fussed over and adorned like the Goddess herself!

The group may then make some final affirmations regarding the power of menstruation and appropriate roles for women to play in today's society. Each participant may also wish to confide her own special ways of honoring her menstrual period. To close, the young woman's mother may give her some jewelry, perhaps a family heirloom piece, or anything featuring red stones. She may also want to formally present her daughter to whatever higher power they recognize, asking for protection and guidance.

When the ritual ends, feasting begins. Red foods represent fertility; guests may wish to toast the young woman with red wine. Perhaps other family members will choose to participate at this point. Men often find it hard to stay away during the ceremony and are very pleased when finally welcomed to join the festivities. Above all, this ritual should be exactly as the young woman wants it, so that she may discover a new degree of trust in her body and in herself.

If such a formal ritual seems too complex or inappropriate for your family, simple variations are fine. One mother told her daughter that when she got her period, she could choose any three things to do in celebration. On the first day of her menarche, she opted for: 1) a shopping trip; 2) total silence from Mom for the entire day; 3) a steak. The last was somewhat controversial for this vegetarian family, but as her mother observed, "Eating a steak was my daughter's ultimate statement of adult decision-making power."

Another option is for mother and daughter to go off together to some favorite outdoor place, connecting with nature and each other. They may go hiking or canoeing, or perhaps build a campfire together, as long as they spend time alone and make it a celebratory day. The mother could use this time to review her daughter's birth and childhood, with stories of what she was like when she was younger, and all the great things she has done in her life thus far. She might also share her visions and her hopes for her daughter's future.

In addition to the aforementioned gift of jewelry, some mothers allow their daughters to pierce their ears on this day, presenting them a gift of earrings with red stones. Another precious keepsake is a "Menarche Book," comprised of photos of all the women in the family (suitable for passing on to the next generation).

The day could end with the mother drawing a bath for her daughter, perhaps placing flower petals on the water. When it is over, the two can decide how to share the news with the rest of the family, and whether a special event of some kind is desired. Again, the most important thing is the young woman's comfort; if she happily participates in planning a larger celebration, she will joyfully remember it for the rest of her life.

Reprinted from *The Women's Wheel of Life: Thirteen Archetypes of Woman at Her Fullest Power*, by Elizabeth Davis and Carol Leonard

Dancing with
Our Hormones

Sometime in my early twenties, I remember wondering why female animals went into heat while we women apparently did not. How could this universal fact of mammalian sexuality be omitted from the most highly evolved species? Some scientists conjectured that the intellectual aspect of human desire had long ago preempted any underlying biological patterns. Yet this did not explain my own fluctuations of desire, seemingly unrelated to person, mood, or setting. Lacking any leads for the time being, I put my question on hold.

The turning point in my inquiry came after the birth of my second child. It was time to resume the use of birth control, and having tried almost every method available with minimal degrees of satisfaction, I decided to learn about fertility awareness. I soon discovered why postpartum women are often discouraged in this pursuit. Because I was breast-feeding and not yet menstruating, my hormone levels fluctuated daily and my fertility signals were all over the spectrum. But after months of observation, I began to catch on. Once I reestablished my cycle, I observed the signs and symptoms of my fertility not only in mucus changes and basal temperature fluctuations but also in the sexual mood swings that accompanied these. Beyond a doubt, I saw that my desire for sex was greater when I was fertile. I also noticed that I made copious amounts of slippery secretion mid-cycle, which made lovemaking easy and seemed to stimulate both me and my partner with a distinctive, erotic scent. Perhaps, I thought, we women have a "heat" of our own after all!

I recall attending a midwifery conference some years ago, when a physician (one of the few male presenters) mentioned in passing that according to his patients, the ovulatory phase was the time they felt most like making love. "How about the only time!" one of the women in the audience piped up, and the entire room broke into laughter. A moment of truth, it seems, and in marked contrast to the "anytime, ever ready" notion perpetuated by the media.

Since then, numerous studies have focused on women's hormones and how they affect health, personality, behavior, and sexual response. Let's look at these key hormones, consider their actions in detail, then explore the delicate choreography of their effects within the monthly cycle.

The Hormones

What, exactly, are hormones? The word *hormone* comes from the Greek *horman*, which means to arouse, excite. Hormones are secreted by certain tissues in the body and travel via the blood or other fluids to other tissues, which they stimulate in particular ways. We used to think there was a difference between the hormones and the neurotransmitters—the chemicals that allow brain cells to communicate—but now we know that hormones also trigger activity in the brain.

Even more interesting is the fact that hormones are not nearly as specific in origin as we once thought. For example, estrogen, considered the quintessential female hormone, is made primarily by the ovaries under signals from the pituitary gland, which is further regulated by the hypothalamus. However, estrogen is also made and utilized by the bones and the blood.

Estrogen plays a major role during puberty, causing breast development, changes in sweat glands that produce body odor, changes in the vagina and its secretions, and enlargement of the external genitals (labia and clitoris). In a sexually mature woman, estrogen triggers ovulation, and during pregnancy it is responsible for breast growth, vaginal and cervical changes, and uterine enlargement.

Progesterone is another key hormone in women's lives. It is produced by the ovaries, specifically by the disintegrated egg follicle known as the corpus luteum, and also plays a role in the monthly cycle. Once ovulation has occurred, progesterone keeps the uterine lining growing so that it can sustain the embryo in the event of conception. During pregnancy, it reduces uterine irritability so the uterus will retain its contents. Eventually, the placenta takes charge of its manufacture.

Now let's see how these hormones work in concert during an average cycle of twenty-eight days. On day one, as menstruation begins, one of the pituitary hormones, follicle-stimulating hormone (FSH), begins to surge. It triggers the ovaries to start producing estrogen. Around day five, estrogen enters the bloodstream and flows to the pituitary gland. When estrogen reaches a certain level, the pituitary secretes less FSH and releases another hormone, luteinizing hormone (LH).

The Menstrual Cycle

▬▬▬ estrogen	– – ·– –	FSH (follicle stimulating hormone)
– – – – progesterone	●–●–●–●	Basal body temperature
▬▬▬ LH (luteinizing hormone)		

This brings us to mid-cycle, or day fourteen. Estrogen is at its peak, and LH flows to the ovary to stimulate one of the follicles there to ripen and release an egg. The egg bursts from the follicle and is drawn into the fallopian tube: this is ovulation. Once empty, the follicle becomes the corpus luteum and starts to produce progesterone.

Please refer to the diagram on the previous page. Note that estrogen levels peak mid-month, just as progesterone levels are beginning to rise.

Progesterone reaches its peak around day twenty-four or twenty-five; at this point, if fertilization has not occurred, LH shuts down, the corpus luteum withers, and progesterone levels drop sharply. Meanwhile, estrogen levels will have gradually reached their lowest point as well; when both have hit bottom, menstruation occurs.

Another hormone that fluctuates regularly in our bodies is testosterone, produced by the adrenal glands (as one of the family of androgens) and also by the ovaries. Testosterone levels in women are seldom more than a tenth of those in most men, except during pregnancy if a woman is carrying a male fetus. Testosterone peaks twice within the monthly cycle, once with ovulation and again with menstruation.

Then there is oxytocin, another hormone produced by the pituitary. Oxytocin is generated both cyclically and in response to certain emotional stimuli. Among other things, it contracts the uterus and is thus elevated immediately before and during menstruation. It also spikes with orgasm and childbirth. It has been found to enhance fertility in women by increasing movement of the fallopian tubes, and to increase the sperm count in men when given by nasal spray. More on this fascinating hormone in a moment.

Perhaps the "mother of all hormones" is DHEA, as it can be transformed by the body into any other sex hormone. Like testosterone, it is a steroid hormone, made primarily by the adrenals but also by the ovaries. Although DHEA cycles throughout the day, it has no particular correlation to the menstrual cycle. It is thought to be responsible for mediating the ebb and flow of other sex hormones, lending continuity to sexual behavior and communication. DHEA is present in all mammals, but humans are unique in that levels are equal in males and females. This may partially explain the more continuous sexual receptivity of women as compared to that of other mammals.

Physical Changes Throughout the Cycle

Now that the key hormones are in place, let's look at their effect on us at different points in the cycle. Keep in mind that the twenty-eight-day cycle is fairly common but far from standard; cycles may run as short as twenty-one days or longer than forty. Fluctuations in cycle length from month to month are also normal.

Menstruation itself may last as few as three days or as many as seven. Women with longer periods often have a break in the middle when the flow stops before resuming for a day or two. Immediately after menstruation ends, most women have several days with little or no vaginal secretion. The fertility-awareness method calls these dry days, which are generally safe from risk of conception—but if you want to make love during this time, you need ample stimulation to lubricate. Depending on how long menstruation lasts and the overall length of the cycle, dry days may be numerous or entirely absent. How so? Take a look at the chart on page 45, which compares the cycles of several different women. Note that regardless of overall cycle length, ovulation occurs fourteen days before menstruation begins. Barring disease or other abnormal conditions, this time span is biochemically fixed. Variation occurs only in the preovulatory phase, where length of menstruation and the number of both dry and preovulatory days may be somewhat unpredictable.

Sample Menstrual Cycles

◎

Average/Long Cycle	Short Cycle	Stress-affected Cycle
Day/Discharge	*Day/Discharge*	*Day/Discharge*
1 menses	1 menses	1 menses
2 menses	2 menses	2 menses
3 menses	3 menses	3 menses
4 menses	4 spotting	4 spotting
5 menses	5 menses	5 dry
6 spotting	6 menses	6 dry
7 dry	7 spotting-slick	7 slippery
8 dry	8 slick	8 moist
9 dry	9 stretchy	9 moist
10 dry	10 dry	10 damp
11 dry	11 dry	11 dry
12 dry	12 dry	12 dry
13 creamy	13 dry	13 stretchy
14 creamy	14 dry	14 slippery
15 wet-milky	15 dry	15 wet
16 slippery	16 dry	16 dry
17 stretchy	17 gummy	17 dry
18 dry	18 gummy	18 dry
19 gummy	19 dry	19 pasty
20 dry	20 slippery	20 gummy
21 pasty	21 damp	21 dry
22 pasty	22 menses	22 dry
23 gummy	23 dry	
24 dry	24 dry	
25 dry	25 dry	
26 dry	26 dry	
27 dry	27 dry	
28 damp-spotting	28 menses	
29 slick		
30 menses		

Preovulatory days are characterized by a buildup of white and creamy vaginal secretion. Gradually, this is replaced by a clear, slippery, and profuse fertile mucus, which looks something like egg whites. Ovulation takes place when fertile mucus reaches peak levels, at which time it has a unique quality known as "spin" (from the German *spinnbarkeit*). If you take a bit of it between your fingers and then pull your fingers apart, it will stretch to form a strand. This mucus has the same alkaline pH as seminal fluid and the perfect molecular structure for sperm to swim through. It can also keep sperm living in the vagina for up to five days. This is why, when using fertility awareness as a contraceptive method, you must abstain or use protection at the first sign of secretion after your dry days. You never know when your mucus will shift to fertile, and when it does, any sperm in the vaginal canal or cervical crypts (small pockets within the cervical opening) can be kept viable until an egg is released.

Fertile mucus is present for approximately five to seven days, then it shifts abruptly to a drier, stickier, yellow-white secretion. Nevertheless, a woman is not safe from risk of conception until three and a half of these postovulatory days have passed, allowing time for the more acidic pH of this mucus to kill off any remaining sperm. In a twenty-eight-day cycle, this brings us to about day nineteen or twenty.

The rest of the month is characterized by the same stickier mucus—with one exception. Just before menstruation begins, some women note a secretion that closely resembles fertile mucus. This is actually a mucus plug from the cervix, which has served to protect the uterus from infection. It is shed spontaneously as progesterone levels fall, at which point menstruation is set to begin.

An important aside: it takes time—at least six months of careful observation—to know enough about your cycle to be able to use fertility awareness as a contraceptive method, or to use a barrier method only when at risk of pregnancy. It is easy to get confused in the beginning. Fertile mucus looks very much like arousal lubrication. Infection can also alter the appearance of vaginal and cervical secretions. Allow enough time to get to know what is normal for you so that you readily perceive these variations.

Besides changes in secretion, women also experience fluctuations during the cycle in breast size, weight, pelvic sensations, and body temperature. Mid-cycle, breast tenderness and enlargement are due to water retention, which may also cause a pound or two of weight gain. (As estrogen levels fall, these effects diminish.) Also noteworthy is the mid-cycle sensation of *mittelschmerz*, which may range from a subtle twinge to a strong cramping feeling as the egg is released from the ovary.

Breast and weight changes later in the cycle are partially due to a second peak of estrogen and are further exaggerated by the increasing presence of progesterone. Progesterone is known as a heat-producing hormone, and high levels may cause a noticeable rise in body temperature. In contrast, when levels plunge premenstrually, women typically experience cold hands and feet.

There are other physiological changes that account for the usual premenstrual symptoms. High levels of androgens may cause intestinal cramping or diarrhea; conversely, some women experience constipation in this phase. Androgens also cause expansion and constriction of blood vessels; as levels fluctuate, women may experience headaches, inflammation of varicose veins, or a rapid heartbeat.

A common question of women in their mid-thirties is why PMS seems to be getting worse, or if never a problem before, suddenly noticeable for the first time. As we age, the mid-cycle estrogen peak soars higher, while the second rise tends to diminish. With less estrogen in the luteal phase, effects of progesterone and the androgens become more exaggerated. Very young women tend to experience similar effects but for a different reason—because their bodies are still maturing, they have less estrogen to modify relatively high testosterone/androgen levels.

During menstruation, progesterone and estrogen are at their lowest levels (although the pituitary gland is primed to release FSH and set the cycle in motion once again). It is interesting that this hormonal low point is literally a fallow phase, a time that allows for rest and rejuvenation both physically and emotionally.

Emotional and Sexual Mood Swings

Perhaps you have already begun to link these physical changes to your own patterns of emotional and sexual response. As menstruation ends and dry days begin, it's no wonder that many women don't feel much like making love. After all, vaginal dryness isn't particularly erotic, and on a purely physical level, the hormonal upswing has just begun. Energetically, though, many women find the preovulatory phase a great time to formulate ideas and make plans, get busy. As estrogen and testosterone increase, the drive is there to get things done.

Accordingly, ovulation is the high point of the month, a time of peak performance. A woman's skill at manipulating small objects increases dramatically as her estrogen levels rise.[1] Numerous studies have shown that women in their fertile phase turn in top performances in athletic competitions and score higher on achievement and intelligence tests than at any other time of the cycle.[2] The physical effects of the fertile phase—elevated body temperature, fullness and sensitivity of the breasts, the slippery wetness of the vagina as though already aroused—tend to increase women's feelings of vitality, desirability, and self-confidence. All systems are "go" when we are fertile. And like it or not, we are physically "in heat"; if our genitals were exposed and visible to potential partners (rather than being modestly covered up, wiped dry repeatedly, or deodorized with panty liners), telltale signs both visual and olfactory would signal our biological receptivity.

Women unaware of the cycle of mucus changes often think they are developing an infection during the fertile phase. It's not that the secretion is offensive, but it is profuse and tends, when exposed to air and kept warm (as in underwear), to develop a rather musky odor. One woman graphically described this as a "barnyard smell": sweet and somewhat strong. Women's sense of smell is consistently more acute than men's, but at ovulation it is especially sharp and attuned to the classically male musk odor known in its synthetic form as exaltolide. It is a smell most women find quite attractive.

Needless to say, this is a great time for lovemaking. As Sharon says, "It's the time I'm always ready. I don't need foreplay because I'm already wet, but the more I have, the more powerful my orgasm." The intensity of orgasm can be partially correlated to the estrogen peak. A unique propensity of this hormone is to stimulate circulation in the pelvic area, including vaginal tissues. These literally become hot and swollen with blood, and the internal muscles are more sensitive and responsive. The accompanying testosterone peak increases assertiveness and self-confidence, as well as sexual thoughts and fantasies.

Emotionally, a majority of women say they feel decidedly amorous while ovulating. As Sara describes it, "For me, there is both passion and tenderness. I really want Tom, but I don't feel tense or rushed about it. I feel ripe and full, with passion everywhere in my body. I feel like playing and taking my time, because I know I'm geared for maximum sensation and incredible orgasm."

Women typically describe orgasms when fertile as "deep, deep in my vagina," "at the very core of my being," or "a total body experience." One woman adds, "I feel like my whole body, all of me, is one giant sexual receptor." Another states, "I feel sacred when I'm fertile, like all of me is at its best. I feel integrated and very free."

Mary vividly describes both her physical and emotional response as "Sweet . . . like waves of warm honey flowing through me." Another woman notes, "This is the time of the month when I can really move a tremendous amount of energy through my body. Sometimes we make love and I come right away, and I feel let down. But when I'm fertile, there's so much energy already that I can build it up, spread it out, and keep doing that until my orgasm is a total thing, it just carries me off completely." "Totality" and "sweetness" are linked to high estrogen levels. Intense desire for sex, pure lust, correlates to the testosterone peak.

This discussion would not be complete without mentioning the pheromones. These are olfactory stimulants released through the perspiration of both men and women. Pheromones are produced by DHEA, and they appear to act on the brain through a small cavity inside each nostril called the vomero nasal organ. We can't smell pheromones the way we smell flowers, but we register their chemical messages nonetheless. Pheromones are especially concentrated in the armpits and genital area. Estrogen causes pheromones to surge mid-cycle in women.

In 1986, Winnifred Cutler discovered that male pheromones could serve to regulate female menstrual cycles. With just a bit of pheromone essence (collected from male sweat samples) placed under their nostrils, 70 percent of women with irregular cycles became regular in a matter of months. In a similar vein, in 1971, Martha McClintock demonstrated menstrual synchrony among women sharing quarters in college dorms, due to the effects of their pheromones. Even more intriguing is the finding that in monogamous heterosexual couples, sexual rhythms tend to synchronize, with male testosterone surges matching female estrogen and progesterone surges, largely in response to pheromone exposure.[3]

Hormones and pheromones aside, there is yet another aspect to heightened desire at mid-cycle. Particularly in partnerships founded on love, passion may spring from the awareness of our fertility and the knowledge that we have the power to conceive—not necessarily the intent, but the power to re-create ourselves. Listen to what Ellen has to say: "Just knowing I'm fertile gets me completely turned on. This is the time when I most feel the power of creation flowing through me. Once my partner is aware, he intensifies my feelings with his own. We use condoms, and sometimes we 'play the edges' by having long, drawn-out foreplay—there's an element of danger and excitement in being unprotected until we finally get the condom in place. The charge we build up, the intimacy, is really something else!"

For lesbians, synchronous cycling can lead to shared fertile times, with exponentially increased sexual and emotional potential. Meg says, "Sex when we're fertile is a blast, we are both so wet and open, the desire just flows. It is also very emotional at times, so overwhelmingly beautiful that we collapse crying in each other's arms."

The flip side of this passion is the difficulty heterosexual couples may have in using contraception with this awareness, in that it may feel like a violation or, at the very least, a bit of a letdown. Those who use fertility awareness as their only method of contraception either abstain during ovulation or content themselves with sexual activity other than penile-vaginal intercourse. Particularly if a couple has children already and fully understands the potential of this time, or if one wants another child while the other does not, the emotional content of sex mid-cycle can be rather explosive.

We will look more at contraceptive methods and issues later in the chapter. For now, suffice to say that the fertile time is indeed a power point. Apart from sexual activity, some women actually plan key business meetings, important family events, holidays, or new ventures to coincide with this phase. From Gina: "I'd been observing my cycles for a long time, four years maybe, when I finally realized I had more energy and did my best work on the upswing from when my period ended on through ovulation. What's even more interesting is that part of me has incorporated the rhythm of my cycle in my day-to-day planning—I don't even have to think about it anymore."

Does this mean that the postovulatory phase is merely a downhill slide? Not really, for although estrogen diminishes, hormones such as oxytocin and testosterone pick up the slack. It is nonetheless true that progesterone, which reaches a peak about ten days after ovulation, and other substances from the adrenals called aldosterones, have a dampening effect on desire. Christiane Northrup describes the luteal phase as "reflective . . . we turn more inward, preparing to develop or give birth to something that comes from deep within ourselves."[4] Thus women may report less interest in sex in the second part of the cycle.

But several days before menstruation, when progesterone levels decrease and androgens rise again, many women notice another sexual peak. When asked to characterize it, they say, "hot," "intense," "urgent," "driving," or "very physical." Samantha says, "Right before my period, I feel, I don't know, more masculine in my approach to sex, more aggressive." And from Joan: "I want it fast, hot, physically rough. . . . I come quickly, explosively . . . it's great!" Ann observes, "I'm less emotional about sex—really, I just want to get off." Testosterone moves us to pursue, initiate, dominate, with a focus on genital sex.

There is, by the way, an interesting relationship between testosterone and spatial skills, which increase dramatically under its influence.[5] This may explain women's increased tendency at this time to both envision and enact sexual scenarios.

Mild premenstrual symptoms such as heightened sensitivity of the skin, especially the breasts and nipples, may further increase sexual pleasure. Many women prefer being on top at this time so they can control the depth and angle of penetration and the rate of clitoral stimulation. Plus, there is more opportunity in this position for being touched and admired. On the other hand, if premenstrual symptoms are severe, any amount of stimulation may be too much until menstruation is under way.

A few words about PMS. Some experts believe it is caused primarily by low progesterone levels. Insufficient progesterone in the monthly cycle may or may not cause premenstrual irritability but definitely links to episodes of breakthrough bleeding several days before menstruation begins (remember, progesterone's job is to maintain the uterine lining). Increasing numbers of women in my practice report these symptoms occasionally, some chronically. Oddly enough, lab tests don't always corroborate clinical symptoms of deficiency. I speculate that even though progesterone levels appear to be within normal range, they are low relative to the excessively high levels of synthetic estrogens in our bodies. We know that these estrogens have adulterated our food, as various forms of this hormone are used to speed growth and plump up both cattle and chicken. Residues are highly concentrated in eggs, milk, and milk products. An obvious solution is to minimize consumption of these foods or look for organic alternatives.

We are additionally exposed to high levels of xeno-estrogens concentrated in our groundwater. These are derived from the manufacture and breakdown of plastics, pesticides, PCBs, and dioxin. It is difficult to avoid exposure to the xeno-estrogens, which are believed to play a major role in the increasingly early onset of menarche and the rise in breast and prostate cancers. Drinking filtered water, eating food that has been irrigated with pure water as it is grown, and avoiding fish harvested from polluted waters (especially shellfish) can help us avoid exposure. It is also wise to minimize the use of products manufactured with dioxin, a by-product of chemical bleaching used to whiten toilet paper, paper towels, tampons, and other products.[6]

Progesterone administered by vaginal suppository, pill, or cream has been randomly successful at best and may have little more than a placebo effect for conditions other than those cited above. After all, it is the pituitary gland that masterminds ovarian function; it doesn't make sense that dosing the body with hormones would create any lasting effect. A better solution may be found in acupuncture treatment, which can prompt the pituitary gland to release FSH and LH at the right time each month. The ovaries may then begin producing estrogen and progesterone spontaneously, in appropriate amounts.

Another possible cause of PMS may be low serotonin levels in the brain. Serotonin acts as a neurotransmitter, easing connections from one nerve ending to another. It may be easiest to understand the implications of low serotonin by looking at what happens when we have plenty—or too much. Prozac boosts serotonin levels but is also known to decrease sex drive and delay orgasm. Low serotonin levels increase sex drive and make orgasm easy, but very low levels may lead to aggressive, irrational, even violent behavior. Serotonin deficiency in animals induces indiscriminate choice of partner and the compulsion for immediate gratification. Serotonin is also known to diminish with dieting or food restriction (here's a good reason to keep eating premenstrually).[7] It may be possible to treat low serotonin levels nutritionally with the amino acid L-tryptophan. L-tryptophan can be dangerous if taken in excess, but certain foods, such as turkey, have naturally high amounts.

It is fairly easy to correlate emotional responses of moodiness, hysteria, fury, and fear to hormonal shifts around menstruation. But beyond hormonal influences, might there not also be certain psychological precursors to PMS? I recall a client of mine who was quite concerned that she might be pregnant—she was two weeks late and had never missed a period, yet two pregnancy tests came back negative. Several days later she reported this dream: She was in her office, feeling under pressure because of a boom in her business. Her papers began blowing around, all over everywhere; then she heard a voice say,

"Just let go." As it turned out, she actually skipped a cycle completely but then resumed her normal rhythm. Admittedly, this example goes beyond mere PMS, but it illustrates psychological conditions that can cause it to become extreme.

This is a theme I explore at length in my book *Women's Intuition*: the function of the premenstrual phase on a psychic level as a time for letting go, relinquishing control, allowing the end of one cycle to make way for the next. Before sorting and reordering the immediate past or dreaming and developing the next phase must come release, surrender, the death of outmoded views and ways. Consider again the hormonal influences: after progesterone peaks, both it and estrogen plummet, not by gradual decline but in a harrowing fall. Compounding the intensity are increased amounts of testosterone; this hormone spurs us to ruthlessly reexamine hidden parts of ourselves and our significant relationships. Making way for the next round means getting out of the way psychically, bottoming out, returning to one's essence. This is the basis of cyclic renewal.

Depending on how readily or easily this occurs, sex may or may not seem desirable. As Sandra reports, "Once I know my period is going to start—I'm cramping or spotting a little—I like to wait on making love until it really gets going. I feel like keeping to myself until I've turned the corner. It's an energy thing for me." Quite the opposite, Pat reports, "A day or two before my period—wow, look out—I've got only one thing on my mind!"

Even if our premenstrual symptoms are relatively mild and predictable, all of us have a terrible time of it now and then. Screaming at our kids, fighting unrelentingly with our loved ones, breaking or throwing things, crying in public places—these extremes are often the tail end of a very trying, difficult month, or a period of less than optimal health. Poor health and stress definitely disrupt the metabolism and may thus affect hormonal balance. Keeping tabs on ourselves day to day, not overdoing it, and getting enough rest and relaxation all help, but sometimes circumstances call for something more. Take a look at the box on page 75 for special ways to cope.

This brings us to the topic of sex during menstruation, one of our most persistent cultural taboos. Men are still influenced by ancient beliefs that depict association with menstruating women as a brush with the dark side. Old fears run deep—in biblical times menstruating women were considered unclean, as was anything they touched. Even in the last decade, women have been cautioned by physicians that sex at this time might lead to infection, a supposition that has no basis in fact. But under the laws of Moses, sex was strictly forbidden during, and for a week after, the period. Since a woman's primary function at the time was to produce as many children as possible, it's likely her chances were intensified by avoiding her husband until mid-cycle when she was fertile, and when his sperm count had had the opportunity to increase. Christianity upheld these patriarchal strictures; between the eighth and eleventh centuries, laws denied menstruating women access to church facilities. A Scottish medical text of this period admonished:

> Oh! Menstruating woman, thou'rt a fiend
> From which all of nature should be closely screened.[8]

Many indigenous cultures have also isolated menstruating women. Sometimes this has been by women's choice; alternatively, cultural taboos removed women from the rest of society. In her fascinating book *Blood, Bread, and Roses: How Menstruation Created the World*, Judy Grahn suggests that in Neolithic times, menstruating women were isolated (literally sent up a tree) to protect the rest of the tribe, lest the scent of their blood attract predators.[9] And in early patriarchal societies, menstruating women were isolated for being overly powerful and magical: that they could bleed without consequence of illness, debility, or death was utterly confounding and frightening to men. But in matriarchal traditions, the menstrual phase is honored as a time when women unite heavenly and earthly forces: heavenly, in that they link to lunar cycles as they bleed with the moon; earthly, in that they embody cycles of birth, death, and rebirth found in nature. Before the days of tampons or pads, women often let themselves bleed into the earth, and their blood was revered as sacred.

In her wonderful book *Red Flower*, Dena Taylor documents a wide range of women's responses to menstrual symptoms. Particularly noteworthy is the desire for seclusion; many speak of wanting to curl up in bed and relax, sleep by themselves, and avoid going out in public. Some speak of only wanting to be with women, and how nice it would be to have a special place where they could gather with others who are also menstruating.[10] In many indigenous societies, this is the menstrual hut, which symbolizes separation from the ordinary concerns of daily life.

Ernest Hartmann, author of *The Biology of Dreaming*, notes that women dream most between days twenty-five and thirty of the cycle. These dreams are often sexual, aggressive, or even violent, as compared to dreams at ovulation, which tend to be mystical, calming, and more integrative in effect. Dream images during menstruation include speaking animals, animals with men's heads, violent acts, accidents and delays, and broken eggshells, whereas ovulating women report dreams of babies, fragile things, jewels, eggs, exquisite landscapes, and their mothers.[11] In terms of sexual content, women usually dream about having sex with their partner or a close friend when ovulating; when menstruating, it's more often sex with a stranger.

It is the premenstrual phase that is most noted for dreams of death. This makes sense, as it is the lowest point hormonally and the turning point of the cycle as well. When I was still cycling, I was often melancholy at this time of the month—wondering what I would do if one of my children died, or struggling with feelings of despair over difficult situations in my life that I feared would never change. But once I started bleeding, my emotions loosened up and I felt like myself again.

It is important to note that PMS is reportedly more severe when sleep is inadequate. Ernest Hartmann conjectures that women need more sleep at this time for the natural release of dreaming. Note, however, that tranquilizers and sleeping pills sometimes prescribed for PMS may repress or inhibit dreaming.

The Native American tradition holds the dreams of bleeding women in high esteem. Most tribes believe that a girl's dreams at menarche tell of her mission or direction in life. According to Brooke Medicine Eagle, author and shaman, the most astounding prophetic dreams and visions, including those of unimaginable events like the coming of the white man, were brought to the people through the "Moon Lodge," women's ritual place of seclusion during menstruation.[12]

I have come to believe that women's psychic propensity immediately before and during menstruation is primarily linked to the effects of the hormone oxytocin. As mentioned earlier, this hormone also peaks during ovulation, another time women note great clarity and insight in their work and dealings with others. Oxytocin is a unique hormone in that it is released not only by physiological prompting but also in response to certain emotional stimuli. For example, oxytocin causes the vagina to lubricate and the nipples to harden not only with physical contact but at the mere thought of one's lover or of sexual activity. A woman overwhelmed with passion for her partner may have an orgasm the moment she is entered, with very little stimulation. Similarly, breast-feeding mothers reminded of their baby by the cry of another may experience an oxytocin-based let-down of milk by mere thought alone. No wonder oxytocin is called the "love hormone"!

Oxytocin stimulates the release of yet another hormone, vaso-pressin, which increases the potential for deeply meditative theta brainwave states.[13] Thus, women commonly report moments of creative inspiration or insight while making love or in afterglow. In pregnancy, when oxytocin is at an all-time high, women speak intu-itively of knowing their child before it is born, both its gender and its nature. For menstruating women, what society deems raving madness may actually be visionary activity, or at the very least, its potential.

Thus, menstruation affords a cyclic opportunity to explore the Mystery, and perhaps, with the right frame of mind and support, a chance to peer into the future. If you are curious about your dreams at this point in your cycle but generally don't remember them, try keeping paper and pen by the bed. Be sure to record your recollections immediately upon awaking, even if it's four in the morning. Despite what you may think, you won't remember them later.

Women often report yet another peak of sexual activity several days into the menstrual flow. For some, the first two or three days are unap-pealing because of general messiness, but as the flow shifts from heavy to moderate, passion picks up. Says Nancy, "Frankly, I like sex best when I'm having my period. I don't have to worry about birth control (I know my cycle) and I'm in a certain mood—feisty, steamy. I'm prelubricated too, and you know, I don't mind the blood all over every-thing: it's erotic to me and my partner." Or, as Jane says, "I feel free, I feel primal, I feel connected to my power. The blood turns me on: it's a symbol of life, the color of passion." And from Ana: "Actually, I think it's hormones, coming back around, picking up again. I know it's not the usual image, but I feel fresh, renewed. I don't think about the past, I think about the future."

Some experts suggest that taboos on intercourse during menstrua-tion may have been due to women's unbridled libido and increased orgasmic capacity, causing inordinate male attention and resulting social disruption.[14] On the other hand, in Tantric tradition, the most powerful sexual rites require that women be menstruating for the "blending of female red and male white."[15]

Referring to Nancy's statement above, a major area of confusion for many women regards whether or not conception is possible during menstruation. This was one of the questions most often missed by the public on the 1990 nationwide Kinsey Sex Quiz. The correct answer is yes, although rarely does this occur. Our bodies don't menstruate and ovulate simultaneously, but the two can occur back to back. For example, a woman with a twenty-one-day cycle could ovulate as early as day six or seven (remember that the postovulatory phase is fixed at fourteen days). On day five of her menstrual flow, she might already have pre-fertile mucus present that could keep sperm viable until an egg is released a day or two later. Conception before day three is virtually unheard of, particularly when the flow is heavy. Yet fear of pregnancy may prevent women from enjoying the free days that do exist at this time and making the most of them.

This bring us full circle on our hormonal journey, once around a typical cycle. Women suffering from gynecological problems and illnesses have different configurations, though, as do those under the influence of certain contraceptive methods.

Health Problems That Affect the Cycle

Failure to menstruate is called amenorrhea. It may be caused by insufficient body fat, tumors of the hypothalamus or pituitary gland, thyroid disease, diseases affecting the central nervous system, diabetes or other chronic diseases, destruction of the endometrium (uterine lining) by excessive curettage (as used in D&C procedures or abortions), drug or alcohol addiction, adrenal disorders, ovarian cysts, or certain medications. A missed period is occasionally caused by stress or rigorous athletic training.

There are other diseases and conditions that don't always cause amenorrhea but strongly affect the cycle. Endometriosis is fairly widespread and is a major cause of infertility. In women with this condition, for reasons not entirely understood, some portion of the menses flows abnormally up into the fallopian tubes and out the tube ends, and endometrial tissue then embeds or implants either in the tubes or outside on the pelvic organs. These implants continue to go through cyclic changes, but since there is no way for the menses they generate to be shed, they scar over repeatedly until adhesions, or abnormal attachments, begin to form between the pelvic structures. Adhesions may cause the uterus or tubes to twist, may prevent eggs from being released or moved down the tubes, or may lead to the development of ovarian cysts, which ultimately disrupt ovulation.

What causes endometriosis? One explanation is that a cervix that is tightly closed, possibly because of scarring from pelvic infection or traumatic abortion, so interferes with normal menstrual flow that menses escape through the tubes. Symptoms include abnormal bleeding and pain with ovulation, menstruation, intercourse, or bowel movements. Sometimes birth control pills or other medications prove helpful, though alternative treatments of acupuncture, homeopathy, and herbs may work as well or better. Pregnancy may also effect a cure, since the hormonal changes of childbearing tend to shrink the implants down to nothing.

Polycystic ovarian disease, or Stein-Leventhal syndrome, is characterized by major hormonal imbalances and amenorrhea. Low FSH, high estrogen, erratic surges of LH, low progesterone, and elevated male hormones virtually eliminate the cycle.

In this disease, follicles swell but fail to release eggs, then fill with fluid and become cysts. Cells around each egg produce testosterone that converts to estrogen, which fools the body into thinking an egg is ready to be released. The pituitary responds by cutting back on FSH and releasing LH, which normally would cause the egg to break free. But this does not happen; instead, the follicle cyst continues to enlarge. At worst, the cyst might rupture and cause internal bleeding. At the same time, high estrogen levels prevent the uterine lining from shedding, so there are no menses, and this buildup of the endometrium increases the risk of uterine cancer.

How might a woman know she has polycystic disease? Often, the cyst (or cysts) will cause pain or discomfort in the pelvic region. Amenorrhea and abnormal growth of facial or body hair (in response to elevated testosterone) are other telltale signs.

Yet another circumstance that drastically alters a woman's cycle is hysterectomy. In the vast majority of cases, even if the uterus is diseased, the ovaries are fine and can be left in place so that normal hormonal production may continue. If all the reproductive organs are removed, immediate menopause ensues. For further information on complete hysterectomy, see Chapter 7.

Endometrial, cystic, or adenomatous hyperplasia occurs when the normal uterine lining is replaced by an overgrowth of glandular tissue. The overgrowth is caused by high levels of estrogen unbalanced by progesterone—a result of anovulatory cycles. This condition is characterized by irregular and intermittent bleeding, as some parts of the lining behave as though it were day three, others, day twenty-eight, and so on. Most cases of endometrial hyperplasia go away on their own, although a biopsy is recommended to rule out cell abnormality. This condition should definitely be followed closely to make sure it is abating, as women with history of anovulatory cycles have a higher incidence of uterine cancer. Some physicians prescribe progesterone prophylactically (there are also natural progesterone creams). If bleeding becomes chronic, a D&C may help by giving the uterus a fresh start.

Uterine fibroids may also cause bleeding apart from menstruation, making it difficult to track the cycle. Bleeding from fibroids is often correlated to sexual activity. Although fibroids are usually benign, a sonogram to determine their exact size and location is a good idea, particularly if bleeding is excessive. Pregnancy tends to increase the size of fibroids, whereas menopause reduces them. If fibroids grow so large as to impinge uncomfortably on other pelvic organs (one of the largest weighed in at one hundred pounds), surgical removal by myomectomy is an option. Hysterectomy is rarely necessary, and many women with fibroids prefer to wait and see. Dr. Christiane Northrup recommends a three-month trial of a high-fiber, whole-foods diet, eliminating all refined sugar and flour and all dairy products (a potential source of excess estrogen associated with fibroid development). This diet is also recommended for women with endometriosis.[16]

Beyond these conditions, other factors can affect the cycle. Artificial lighting may disrupt lunar regulation of the cycle, particularly if there is a streetlight right outside the bedroom window. Opaque blinds can be used to regulate the amount of light in the room; they should be fully open at the full moon and closed completely at the new moon.

And then there is the busy pace of life, which occasionally turns grueling and causes us to lose our own natural pace and rhythms. We all have personal rhythms, times during the day when we naturally seek food, rest, or stimulation. Some people are morning types, some more nocturnal. Frequently, our personal rhythms are at odds with our social routine; we may not, for example, feel like eating at traditional meal times.

Learning to follow our daily rhythms is important. Many women in my practice have said they would do anything for time alone, a day off once in a while to do exactly as they please. I say, simply make the time, before it is too late! In terms of optimal health, it makes all the difference to follow our most subtle instincts, making sure we have exactly what we want to eat, finding privacy for a few moments when we most need it, or taking a second or two to breathe deeply.

Junk food, stimulants like coffee, sugar, and chocolate, and sedatives like alcohol all obscure our natural biorhythms. This doesn't mean we must give these up completely, but we do need to keep an eye on our intake. These substances tend to stress and debilitate our bodies, causing us to lose needed vitamins and minerals. Moreover, when we are less than healthy, our emotional reactions become extreme, and our abilities to handle life's daily challenges become impaired. Mood elevators like Prozac also interfere with our biorhythms and, if overused, can exacerbate the very emotional problems they are intended to alleviate.

It is unfortunate that most of us know little of the healing properties of tonic and medicinal herbs, but this is relatively easy to remedy. Herbs are allies for health and harmony; when one starts using herbs for self-improvement, desires for harmful substances or less-than-healthful foods often begin to fall away. There are many fine beginning texts on herbology; explore them at your local bookstore or library.

The Effects of Contraceptive Methods

No discussion of contraception is complete without mention of safe sex as a means to protect ourselves from hepatitis B and C, HIV, and other sexually transmitted diseases. Although condoms and latex dams are simple enough in concept, some women have difficulty insisting on their use. This is dangerous, as the incidence of AIDS is rising most dramatically among women, particularly heterosexual women.

The need to take last-minute precautions changes sexual dynamics, particularly those of foreplay. Ideally, a couple should discuss safe sex in advance, but often the subject arises concurrently with passion. A number of my clients report being surprised at how bringing up safe sex sets them on equal footing with their male partners: conventional roles of man as aggressive and woman as passive all but wither away. Foreplay then becomes playful, and acts of securing the condom or placing the dam can be humorously erotic.

The Female Condom

Although barrier methods are surveyed later in this section, the female condom bears mention here. This device consists of a sheath of latex with one open and one closed end, each encircled by a rubber ring. The smaller ring (at the closed end) is inserted and placed over the cervix; the larger ring remains outside the body, resting over the labia. Originally developed in Europe, this method has only recently been available in the United States, so we have little data on user satisfaction. Some women report discomfort during intercourse, presumably from the outer ring rubbing against the labia or clitoris—still, the female condom gives a woman the prerogative.

The Pill

Regarding the more popular contraceptive methods, we will start with the birth control pill. Put bluntly, the Pill completely obliterates the cyclical pattern of emotional and sexual response presented earlier in this chapter. The Pill works by effecting a state of pseudo-pregnancy— hormone levels are high enough to trick the body into believing it has already conceived, so ovulation does not occur. Most formulas combine estrogen and progesterone; others use progesterone only (the mini-Pill). An excessive dose of either of these hormones can cause side effects such as weight gain, chronic acne, breast tenderness, nausea, headaches, and fatigue (see chart on page 80). A woman's response to a particular formula is somewhat unpredictable, because much depends on her preexisting balance and sensitivities. This is why a women's health specialist may prescribe as many as five or six brands before her client finds one that is satisfactory.

Whatever the formula, the day-to-day mix is uniform. Thus women on the Pill are hormonally monotone, always the same. Gone are the natural peaks of estrogen, oxytocin, and testosterone. Gone are the creativity and passion of ovulation, the intense, red-hot desire immediately before or during menstruation. Gone too are the psychological benefits of phasing through the cycle, of cyclic completion and renewal. For there is no real menstruation while on the Pill, either; it takes ovulation to trigger the buildup and release of the uterine lining. Pill users have only a little breakthrough bleeding when they have taken the last of the batch and hormone levels drop temporarily. This flow is light and uniform, without variation in length or consistency.

What about sequential, triphasic pills? Don't these attempt to replicate the cycle? Even though triphasic formulas add a bit of progesterone to the latter half of each batch, they nevertheless maintain a predictable pattern, one invariably foreign to a woman's own. When my clients speak of a desire to get off the Pill, they often cite the primary reason as wanting to be more in touch with their bodies. The more we talk, the more it becomes clear that what they really miss is being in touch with themselves, nuances of feeling they once enjoyed, their own unique mind-body blend. It's disturbing to consider the extent to which dosing women with artificial hormones can modify personality and sexual response, but such is clearly the case.

As for the latter, we have ample clinical confirmation of loss of libido in women taking the Pill. Rosemarie Krug, psychobiologist from the Department of Clinical Neuroendocrinology at the Medical University of Lubeck, studied women's responses to erotic imagery, comparing those on the Pill to those who were not. Three times a month—at ovulation, premenstrually, and at menstruation—study participants were shown a series of rapid images of naked men, babies, and women combing their hair, and were asked to categorize their response as sexual, maternal, or body-related. Women at ovulation were much quicker to spot the babies and naked men and to read sexual connotations into hair-care images than were women on the Pill, whose responses were at a low ebb throughout the month, never reaching the intensity of normally cycling women. Krug concluded that the Pill negatively affects libido by lowering testosterone levels and obliterating natural hormonal peaks at ovulation.

Yet another study explored the effects of male pheromones on women using the Pill with those who were not. A number of male participants were asked to wear the same T-shirt for several days without showering or using deodorants or cologne; they could not smoke or eat spicy foods. The T-shirts were put into boxes for the women to smell and rate according to appeal. Women not on the Pill were most attracted by the scent of men with immune systems complementary to their own, which researchers concluded would naturally benefit their offspring. But women on the Pill chose men that had immune systems almost identical to their own. Researchers concluded that women on the Pill behaved as though they were pregnant, choosing men more like kin for the sake of protection, rather than men suitable for mating.[17]

I find the implications of this study to be most significant. These effects of the Pill may be less of an issue for the woman already in a relationship, but for the woman still looking for Mr. Right, it's disturbing to think that the Pill could prevent her from recognizing him at a crucial biological level.

The Pill may be therapeutic for certain gynecological problems such as endometriosis or pathologically painful menstruation, but we must remember that relief obtained in these cases merely masks underlying causes. Again, acupuncture (along with dietary changes) may effectively reeducate the system to a more balanced hormonal state.

Acupuncture may also be useful for women coming off of the Pill. It is not uncommon for women to miss a period or two when they first stop taking the Pill, as the body has forgotten what to do and needs to get back on track. If the rhythm is lost for six months or more, acupuncture and herbs can stimulate pituitary secretion of LH and FSH, with subsequent ovarian response. This treatment is definitely preferable to the use of Clomid, a potent fertility drug notorious for causing multiple pregnancies. Problems with delayed cyclical function are much more common after the age of thirty—ironically, a time when women often quit the Pill specifically to get pregnant. Herbal tinctures of vitex and cottonroot bark may be helpful.

The IUD

Although the intrauterine device is rarely used today, let's consider its effects on a woman's cycle. With the exception of the Progestasert, the IUD does not directly alter hormonal balance. However, many women using IUDs report heavier and more painful periods than before. Originally, women getting an IUD were told that these problems were merely mechanical—that the device caused low-grade irritation sufficient to prevent pregnancy but with side effects of cramping and increased bleeding. What they were not told is that the IUD does not prevent conception; it merely prevents implantation of the already fertilized ovum. After all, there is no mechanical barrier to prevent the sperm from meeting the egg. The so-called heavy periods with the IUD are often spontaneous miscarriages, month after month after month.

Thus the hormonal effects of the IUD, though indirect, are quite drastic. If conception occurs, dramatic changes in the levels of estrogen and progesterone follow. I recall piecing this realization together many years ago while wearing an IUD; I couldn't wait to get it out! The idea of miscarrying repeatedly as a method of contraception was both physically and spiritually repugnant to me. I know that some women continue to use the IUD and consider it a godsend. But the problems associated with its use are far from minor, including infertility from uterine scarring, tubal pregnancy, and tubal rupture.

The Progestasert device is a bit different. It works something like the mini-Pill: elevated levels of progesterone tend to prevent eggs from maturing and chemically alter the cervical mucus to make it inhospitable to sperm. However, the device commonly causes menstrual irregularities, such as prolonged bleeding and occasional amenorrhea.

Norplant and Depo-Provera

There are two other progesterone-based methods of contraception currently available. Norplant, inserted in the arm, provides up to five years' protection from pregnancy by slowly releasing progesterone into a woman's bloodstream. Depo-Provera is injected every three months. The main difference between these two is the amount of progesterone—Norplant levels are similar to those of the mini-Pill, but Depo-Provera is very high-dose. Accordingly, side effects from Depo-Provera are more extreme: cessation of menses, weight gain, breast tenderness, depression that may persist for many months after discontinuation, bone density decrease when used over long periods of time, and dramatic reduction of high-density lipoprotein cholesterol (the good kind, which keeps blood cholesterol levels low). Norplant side effects include menstrual irregularities similar to those of the mini-Pill, and a tendency to develop ovarian cysts.

Tubal Ligation

The nearly foolproof method of tubal ligation, long touted as having virtually no side effects, merits closer investigation. Studies have shown a correlation with menstrual cycle disruption, and in rare cases, early menopause. Progesterone levels are known to decrease for six months to a year after the procedure, contributing to severe PMS. Sometimes, levels never return to normal.[18] Still, this is definitely the right choice for some women.

The Diaphragm and the Cervical Cap

What about the barrier methods? Clearly, these have no physiological effect on a woman's cycle. But the minor inconveniences are considerable, including chemical irritation from spermicide, lack of spontaneity, messiness, and reduced sensation.

My extensive experience with the cervical cap (I ran an FDA approved study from 1982 to 1986) has led me to favor it over other barrier methods. Compared to the diaphragm, it uses very little spermicide: no additional applications are required for repeated intercourse. It can be left in place for several days and is small enough to be virtually undetectable. A little-known fact about the diaphragm is that although it feels snug when first placed, the vagina expands so much with arousal that even an oversized fit will move and slide around freely during intercourse, readily admitting seminal fluid. Thus the jelly inside the diaphragm becomes so diluted that more must be added before having sex again, in an attempt to catch the sperm before they get over the rim. In contrast, the cap fits over the cervix securely with suction, forming a stable mechanical barrier. In addition, when the user is fertile, the cap retains her alkaline fertile secretions so that her vagina stays naturally acidic and inhospitable to sperm (seminal fluid is also alkaline). Thus the cap works with a woman's chemistry rather than against it; it is more truly a barrier method than the diaphragm, which relies largely on spermicide for its effectiveness.

A bonus of cap use is increased familiarity with your cycle; it is easy to see what phase you are in depending on the type of secretion your cap collects. Also, women who use the cap report fewer yeast and other vaginal infections than women using the diaphragm, since chemical disturbance of vaginal flora is virtually nonexistent.

Having personally used a diaphragm for fourteen years, I know well the frustrations of nagging discomfort and disrupted spontaneity associated with its use. There were many occasions when I was tempted to leave the diaphragm in the drawer, or just toss it in the trash. Eventually I realized that much of my resistance was due to reduced levels of sensation while making love. Around this time, news of the G-spot hit the press, and suddenly it all made sense. By virtue of its design, the front rim of the diaphragm must displace the G-spot in order to lodge behind the pubic bone. No wonder I couldn't feel much! Once I learned fertility awareness and could safely use a diaphragm only when necessary, my suspicions were confirmed. When I switched to the cap, the problem was solved completely, as the cap sits way back in the vagina, nowhere near the G-spot.

As mentioned earlier, some women use fertility awareness as birth control and simply abstain during the ovulatory phase. This may cause considerable frustration, though, as the intense desire when fertile must consistently be ignored or expressed in ways other than vaginal-penile intercourse. Women in my practice increasingly choose to combine fertility awareness with a barrier method.

Many alternate their use of the cap or diaphragm with having their partner use condoms. They say it feels good to share the responsibility, switching back and forth from month to month, or from time to time. A comment from Suzanne: "My partner and I had run the gamut in birth control, and we ended up with barrier methods for safety's sake. But it didn't feel right to me to always be the one who had to remember, to take charge. It's nice when my partner takes his turn with a condom: I can just sit back and relax, and I like the feeling of my body being completely natural. It helps me enjoy sex more."

Hormonal Changes by Decade

Thus far, we've explored the sexual mood swings of the monthly cycle in somewhat generic terms. However, the hormonal balances we typically run in our twenties are quite different from those in our thirties or forties—each decade has its own sexual flavor. Later chapters will explore the evolution of our sexuality in the context of maturation. For now, here is an overview of the hormonal underpinnings of these changes.

The Twenties

Women are more physiologically stable in their twenties than in their teens. Testosterone and estrogen surges have leveled off somewhat, although estrogen levels remain high. At this age, many women tend to feel more sexually receptive than assertive and may be attracted to strong and dominating partners more often than they care to admit. Social factors figure strongly here, in that young women in the prime of their reproductive capacity need care and protection in order to raise their young. It is unfortunate that in our culture, this need is not mediated by the love and support of female family members and peers, which might allow a young woman to more selectively choose her mate.

High levels of estrogen also move women at this age to seek intimacy, which can be difficult to find with men their own age, who are strongly testosterone-driven and thus more inclined to sexual conquest than genuine closeness. But women need intimacy—not only for emotional reasons, but for biological ones. The acts of touching, kissing, and caressing prompt the release of oxytocin, which triggers a mutual bonding response. Thus, women in their twenties long more for passionate, ecstatic touch than raw sex, precisely for the opportunity it affords for bonding.

PMS can be a problem at this age if a woman is less than conscious of its effects, particularly if she is living with a partner who must now deal with these effects, too.

The Thirties

The decade of the thirties is one when women begin to come into their sexual power. It is also the time of life most noted for overwork, one when the average woman feels she runs all day and never quite catches up. Stress may cause DHEA levels to drop, which can lead to decreased levels of testosterone, less pheromone production, reduced sex drive, and less orgasmic capacity. Stress may also precipitate some wicked PMS, which may already be a problem as less estrogen is being produced in the luteal phase to buffer the effects of progesterone and the androgens.

But if stress can be managed or set aside, testosterone levels continue to rise. This can boost a woman's confidence, leading her to worldly success and greater sexual assertiveness than ever before. Orgasm is very important to women in their thirties! They are now more active than receptive, more sure of their needs and intent on satisfaction.

The Forties

For many women, there comes a time in their early forties when PMS takes on new character, apart from stress. As we approach menopause, occasional anovulatory cycles cause our hormones to surge, in order to force ovulation to continue. This results in much higher levels of estrogen and progesterone than usual, causing extreme heights and also depths as levels drop before menstruation.

Testosterone also continues to increase, leading women to be more sexually experimental and aggressive than ever before. Woman reach their sexual peak sometime in their forties, much as men do in their late teens/early twenties. This discrepancy may prompt some heterosexual women to seek younger partners; others find that partners their own age complement them perfectly. Men in their forties experience a decline in testosterone, which unmasks estrogen, leading them to be more touch-oriented, sensitive, and receptive than when they were younger.

The Fifties

The average age of menopause is fifty-two, but women may enter menopause much earlier, even in their late thirties. As menopause approaches, it causes major shifts in the cycle as levels of estrogen, progesterone, testosterone, and other hormones fluctuate daily, much as in adolescence. Missed periods, longer-than-usual periods, and scant, irregular bleeding are all considered normal at this time. As women begin to leave the monthly cycle behind, they experience dramatic mood swings and fluctuating sexual desires (again, much as in adolescence).

* * *

In the next chapter, we will look specifically at sex in the child-bearing cycle, including the fertility dance leading to conception. Particularly if a woman knows her cycle and recognizes her fertility signals, she will be likely to experience conception as it occurs. We will also consider how out-of-sync desires for conception between partners can affect the tone, ease, and frequency of sexual sharing in relationship.

Ways to Cope with PMS

1. Evoke your emotions. Listen to the most sentimental, moving music you can find, the kind that hits the spot, and let yourself cry, yell, rave if you will. We midwives tell new mothers that letting their tears flow will help their milk come down; the same is true of tears and menstruation.

2. Experience the dark side. Review the underbelly of the month, all the things that have hurt you, made you blue, made you feel powerless or furious. Be aware of accumulated tensions in your psyche and your body.

3. Note spontaneous resolutions. As you relive the negative events of your last cycle, note any inspirations for doing it differently or better next time, any resolutions. This is a great time for saying, "I'm never going to let ___ happen to me again," or, "I'm not going to do ___ anymore!"

4. Eat. Studies have shown that as naturally as women gain a few pounds before menstruating, they lose them immediately after. In one such study, the control group struggled not to respond to food cravings. They didn't gain weight, but they didn't lose weight once menstruation was over, either. You need more calories at this time. Many women report cravings for green vegetables, as well as foods high in calcium and protein, which can balance chocolate and sugar splurges that provide only a temporary lift.

5. Exercise. A full-body, aerobic routine is especially good pre-menstrually. Aerobic exercise stimulates circulation and

elimination, thus counteracting symptoms like backache, bloating, cramping, and fatigue.

6. Stay warm. To compensate for circulatory changes, stay cozy. Wear socks, wrap up in a blanket, take a sauna, turn up the heat, and wear loose, nonconstricting clothing (no tight jeans, tight shoes, tight bras, etc.).

7. Make space for yourself. Take time off, find ways to defer your responsibilities, or duck out of them completely if they are truly excessive. Clear the decks! And make time to be alone, do the things that make you feel good. In a word, indulge.

8. Have sex if you want to. A little sex goes a long way in alleviating premenstrual tension. But be yourself—weepy, passionate, outrageous, outspoken—and make sex work for you. Masturbate, enjoy your body.

9. Celebrate when your period begins. Do some sort of letting-go-of-the-old ritual: burn letters, discard objects that symbolize entanglement, make affirmations of new beginnings.

Moon Phase Energies and Menstruation

Waxing Moon Menstruation

The waxing moon is a time of growth, of new trends and activities emerging, of new beginnings. This is a time to turn inward and tap your own wisdom, a time to learn new skills and make discoveries.

In Native American culture, the animal of the waxing moon is the raven, who symbolizes exchange of knowledge and flight of the soul. According to the ancient Greeks, the goddess of this phase is Persephone, who walked the underworld.

Full Moon Menstruation

The full moon is outwardly focused: this is a time to bring to bear, to work, and to do. Whereas the waxing moon correlates to daybreak, the full moon is like high noon, a time when things may be revealed. This is a charged phase and a challenging one emotionally, when the dragon nature of menstruating women is fully evident.

In Native American culture, the animal of the full moon is the phoenix, who burns to ashes and then rises anew. The goddess is Ishtar, Red Goddess of Babylon.

Waning Moon Menstruation

The waning moon parallels sunset, when energy subsides and stabilizes. Now is the time to firm up plans, substantiate discoveries, verify knowledge, and let ideas bear fruit.

In Native American culture, the animal of this phase is the she-bear, who signifies the womb and is therefore productive. In ancient Greek culture, the goddess of this phase is Demeter, who signifies the harvest.

New Moon Menstruation

The new moon is inwardly focused and gives us time for contemplation, reflection, and germination. This is the midnight phase, one of rest and recuperation. Subconscious memories and anxieties rise to the surface; significant events are reviewed.

The animal of this phase is the toad: wise, slippery, solitary, and untouchable due to her poisonous exterior. The goddess is the Greek Hecate, the crone, the trickster, the dark one, the reaper.

Adapted from *Dragontime* by Luisa Francia (New York: Ash Tree Publishing, 1988).

Herbs for Menstruation

With all herbs, source and processing make all the difference. Familiarize yourself with any herb farms in your area, and seek out distributors who carry organic products. Good tinctures are dated for reference and generally appear clear, not muddy.

Basil (*Ocimum bascilicum*), particularly the fresh leaf, stimulates bleeding, invigorates, and lifts feelings of depression. A favorite way to take basil is in pesto; served with pasta it is especially good at the onset of menstruation, as the carbohydrates provide calories and warmth.

Catnip (*Nepeta cataria*) is pain-killing, cramp-easing, soothing, and calming. It calms digestive disturbances caused by aldosterones (and is thus renowned for its ability to ease colic in newborns).

Ginger (*Zingiber officinale*) stimulates circulation, warms and balances the body, and also helps dispel gastrointestinal upsets.

Life root (*Senecio aureus*) is best taken by tincture: five to ten drops daily help to regulate the cycle and ease PMS. It may also relieve severe cramps, uterine or intestinal. Herbal lore teaches that life root blossoms were found carefully placed on the oldest grave known.[19] It is especially effective if taken long-term.

Motherwort (*Leonurus cardiaca*) is most effective taken by tincture: take ten drops to relax, fifteen drops to ease menstrual pain. Motherwort is also used for hot flashes during menopause and to ease labor pains.

Nettle (*Urtica dioica*) helps rid the body of excess water, while strengthening the kidneys and adrenals. It also provides vitamin K, carotene, protein, and key minerals for menstruation, such as calcium and iron. It is especially useful for excessive bleeding.

Raspberry (*Rubus species*) is said to represent women's passion and life force. Raspberry tea eases PMS and tones the uterus; it is mood-elevating and elicits, according to Luisa Francia, "passionate menstruation." It is the beverage of choice for women during pregnancy and postpartum.

Rosemary (*Rosmarinus officinalis*), either the oil or leaf, is strengthening and stabilizing to the body. It stimulates bleeding and helps keep energy high and consistent during menstruation.

Estrogen and Progesterone Imbalances

Signs of Estrogen Excess

- nausea and vomiting
- dizziness
- edema
- leg cramps
- increase in breast size
- chloasma (brown pigmentation on face)
- changes in eyesight
- hypertension
- certain headaches (vascular)

Signs of Estrogen Deficiency

- early spotting (days one to fourteen)
- reduced menstrual flow
- nervousness
- painful intercourse due to vaginal changes

Signs of Progesterone Excess

- increased appetite
- tiredness
- depression, mood changes
- breast tenderness
- vaginal yeast infection
- oily skin and scalp
- hirsutism (excess body hair)

Signs of Progesterone Deficiency

- late spotting and breakthrough bleeding (days fifteen to twenty-one)
- heavy menstrual flow, with clots
- decreased breast size

Herbal Sources of Estrogen and Progesterone

Herbs That Stimulate Estrogen Production

- blue cohosh
- black cohosh
- basil
- sage
- black currant
- licorice
- raspberry leaf

Herbs That Stimulate Progesterone Production

- sarsaparilla
- wild yam root
- tansy
- chaste tree (vitex)

The Sexuality of Pregnancy and Birth

Being aware of your monthly cycle may also lead you to notice biological urges for conception. These desires may emerge only in mid-cycle dreams, or you may find yourself fantasizing about babies and birth with increasing frequency. Sometimes, when the desire for a baby has built up over a period of time, women report startling feelings during lovemaking that conception is imminent, regardless of contraceptive precautions. Some report visions of waiting spirits, or images of their infant or toddler to be. As one woman relayed:

> We were in the midst of lovemaking overwhelming from the moment it began, so very powerful, when suddenly I saw this picture in my mind of a blonde, curly-haired little boy and I knew that I could conceive that child, that it wanted to come to me. I tried to tell my partner about it later, but he wasn't ready to hear it—he thought I was fabricating it, I guess. But I never will forget the intensity, the clarity, the ultra-real quality of that moment. From then on, I knew we were destined to have a child together and it was only a matter of time.

No one can really say what brings on such revelations, but they clearly go beyond the physical realm. I think couples deeply in love build up so much intensity in their relationship that it eventually overflows and begins to take form, one way or another. Women speak of this fecund state in somewhat mystical terms. Joanne recalls, "I felt like the veil between worlds, this and another place of souls, began to fall away. Soon, all we had to do was touch, and the awareness of that other place, new life just waiting, was all around us."

Looking back, I can clearly recall the exact moment when each of my three children was conceived. Even now,

> I am surprised by how vivid the memories are, every detail
> of environment and mood crystal clear, my sensory aware-
> ness at its peak. Each time, just moments after orgasm, there
> was a period of truth and realization, extraordinary and
> profound, that left me sure and shaking with the knowledge
> that I was pregnant. There was no turning back: I was forever
> changed!

My experience is somewhat at odds with the notion of "planned pregnancy," which paints conception as a predictable, controllable, matter-of-fact occurrence. According to my midwifery clientele, conception occurs less by deliberation than by surrender. Women commonly report, "Well, this wasn't exactly what we planned—it happened a bit sooner (or later) than we expected, but we were open to it, and we're happy."

For others, it's not so easy. Couples with a history of infertility are often so burdened with anxiety and frustration that lovemaking becomes a chore. If they do conceive, it may take them a while to realize it has finally happened before they can truly relax. Women with a history of traumatic abortions may also have difficulty conceiving and accepting conception once it occurs, particularly if they have not come to terms with previous losses. The same may be true of women who have endured repeated miscarriage, at least until the crucial window of potential repeat has passed.

Sometimes, a woman must face the fact that she stands alone in her desire to conceive. Perhaps she and her partner can't agree on when she should get pregnant, or her partner is having second thoughts about parenthood in general. Frankly, I think we health providers have been remiss in helping women realistically address their biological clock issues. I've had far too many clients in their late thirties or early forties speak wistfully of having children one day when their mate is finally ready or their life is finally in perfect order, only to become severely traumatized when infertility forces them to realize that it's too late.

This confusion regarding appropriate preparation for parenthood is endemic of a society that provides virtually no social or financial support for pregnant women or young families. It also reveals our inculcated quest for perfection, enacted in the endless struggle for material prosperity as prerequisite to happiness. But Mother Nature has other designs. She did not intend us to wait to have children until we've mastered life, or we would have them in our fifties and sixties. Parenting itself is a vehicle for personal growth: it teaches us to love unconditionally, to accept small strides over time, and to make the most of the way things are, rather than longing for perfection. These are important lessons in human maturation, otherwise difficult to come by for those who forego childbearing. But women today who find themselves wanting to have children are often beset with their own doubts, which are magnified by the "rational" reservations of others. This is more than unfortunate. The reproductive impulse is natural, creative, a gift to cycling women—it is friend, not foe. We must reframe and reclaim the inherent power of our ability to conceive!

When conception occurs, a complex series of hormonal, physical, and psychological changes begin to take place. These changes profoundly affect a woman's emotional stability and sense of self. Especially at first, pregnancy can make a woman feel like her life has been turned on end. But this is normal; it is part of the process.

Pregnancy is comprised of three trimesters, each lasting approximately thirteen weeks. Each of these trimesters has its own challenges and joys, which begin to make sense when the process is viewed as a whole.

The First Trimester

◎

Even though women seldom show their pregnancy in the first trimester, dramatic changes are taking place. When conception occurs, progesterone and estrogen levels do not drop as in the monthly cycle but rise to several times the normal amounts. This causes sweeping changes to occur throughout the mother's body. Her thyroid gland enlarges, which raises her metabolic rate to provide the energy needed for fetal development and other physiological demands of pregnancy. Her blood vessels dilate to allow for increased blood volume. Her adrenals produce additional aldosterone to counter the sodium loss that would otherwise occur with increased estrogen and progesterone. The latter may explain why she may feel less sexual than usual at the beginning of pregnancy, at least for the first few weeks.

But this is not the only reason her desire may be waning. Morning sickness, which occurs as her body adjusts to elevated hormone levels, is hardly conducive to cuddling and carrying on. In fact, she may feel exceedingly vulnerable at this stage and may need lots of nurturing from her partner. Simple acts of kindness, like being brought some toast first thing in the morning, mean more to her than comfort alone; they are a measure of her partner's commitment, and as such can lead to increased intimacy once nausea is overcome.

Other physical changes affect the breasts, particularly the nipples, which become hypersensitive to touch. As Alicia reports: "My breasts are rather small and I'm not that confident about them, but when I'm pregnant, they become a focus in our lovemaking." Cheryl sums it up succinctly: "My partner and I have never gotten more pleasure from my breasts than when I was pregnant."

Another inconvenience of early pregnancy is frequent urination, due to uterine enlargement and pressure on the bladder. However, increased circulation in pelvic tissues at this time as a means for uterine growth can also lead to pelvic engorgement, similar to that in premenstrual or ovulatory phases of the cycle. This may cause a woman to desire deep and forceful penetration, which many women worry might not be safe. There has been much debate on this subject over the years; notions that intercourse and orgasm have deleterious effects on mother and baby have come and gone. For a while, physicians advised that orgasm be strictly avoided, as the resulting uterine activity might cause oxygen deprivation for the baby. However, although there is no doubt that orgasm causes uterine contractions, they are too minor to have any serious effect on placental circulation. Additionally, increased heart rate and deeper breathing tend naturally to compensate for any adverse effects.

There have also been moralistic admonitions against "exposing the fetus to an atmosphere of carnal desire." Let's hope that one is behind us! Some studies link uterine and fetal infection to intercourse in the last trimester, but findings are inconclusive due to variables of stress level, dietary habits, and preexisting health conditions.

On the other hand, if there is a history of miscarriage or episodes of bleeding in the current pregnancy, sexual activity should probably be curtailed, at least for the first trimester. It is important to remember, though, that one in four women have some bleeding in early pregnancy, yet only one in ten miscarry. Particularly if bleeding coincides with the time of the month menstruation would ordinarily occur, there is less cause for concern. In this case, it seems that the body maintains its old rhythm for a while until new hormonal levels are established.

If there is a history of premature labor or birth, sexual activity may be forbidden later in pregnancy, depending on whether the cervix shows any signs of premature softening or opening. Sometimes a woman must stay in bed for some time until her baby is ready to be born, with intercourse and orgasm strictly taboo.

Barring these exceptions, sex brings the physiological benefits of increased pelvic circulation, release of tension, and internal muscle toning particularly helpful in preparation for birth. There are immense psychological benefits, too, which help mediate the scope and speed of change. Many couples describe their sexual encounters in pregnancy as rebonding experiences, akin to those in the initial phase of their relationship. No wonder, for both partners are assuming new roles and discovering certain aspects of each other heretofore unknown. For heterosexual couples, there is the extra boost of not having to think about birth control.

A woman's level of desire in the first trimester may also be related to the sex of the child she is carrying. At about six to eight weeks, when the baby's brain is developing, male fetuses are exposed to an enormous dose of testosterone, the level of which is four times that of infancy and childhood.[1] This undoubtedly has some effect on the mother, quite possibly increasing her libido. By the same token, a mother's ability to recognize the sex of her unborn might have a hormonal basis, since surges of testosterone continue to occur in male fetuses at regular intervals during gestation.

Precisely how the effects of early pregnancy influence a woman's sexuality depends also on her personality, her self-esteem, her desire for the baby, the stability of her primary relationship(s), and various other psychosocial factors. Often, women in our culture feel somewhat frightened upon confirmation of pregnancy—excited, but apprehensive nonetheless. This is a normal reaction, considering that most of us know little or nothing about childbearing until pregnant, most of us have never witnessed a birth, and many have not even held a baby. Despite the thrill of being pregnant, many women feel considerable anxiety about joining the ranks of our least acknowledged and most underprivileged social group: mothers. A newly pregnant woman soon learns that society considers motherhood a personal venture that must somehow be done "on the side," squeezed onto an already loaded palette of responsibilities. Thus, it is never too early to begin the work of establishing a support system, whether by getting together with other expectant mothers or by forging new alliances with female relatives.

Women's reactions to the specific stages of childbearing also vary according to personality type. A physically oriented woman, for example, may find the natural softening of her body and loss of emotional control caused by hormone swings at the onset of pregnancy to be excruciating. She is apt to complain that her body doesn't work anymore; no longer can she make her way by physical intent alone. Naturally, this will affect her sexual self-image. For her, the key to adjustment is to express her feelings, while learning more about the unique capabilities of her changing body.

More emotionally oriented women are quite the opposite, glorying in the heightened sensitivities of pregnancy. They may enjoy sex as much as ever, as long as there are no major upheavals in their relationship. Increased needs for food and exercise may go unnoticed, though, resulting in decreased physical energy and emotional instability, which ultimately affects sexual enjoyment. Emotionally based women must learn to set aside their feelings occasionally to focus on messages from their bodies. They also need concrete, factual information on nutrition and the physiology of pregnancy to offset some tendency to fanaticism.

Mentally oriented women, with a penchant for control and having everything in place, may make their adaptation by the book and yet feel disoriented by surges of emotion and extreme mental states beyond their experience. They must find a way to explore their feelings, perhaps by connecting mind and body through dance, movement, massage, or whatever serves to facilitate spontaneity and discovery of the inner voice. This can add an entirely new dimension to sexual experience.

An oft-underrated aspect of pregnancy is the sweeping effect of elevated hormones on the psyche. Or perhaps we get only the downside, the negative view that paints expectant mothers as borderline crazies—forgetful, hopelessly moody, and foolishly preoccupied. It is clear that our culture considers pregnant women childlike, dolling them up in puffed sleeves with little-girl prints. But let's listen to what pregnant women themselves have to tell us about their psychological state: "I've never felt better in my life," or, "I feel fulfilled, like I'm really myself at last." Consider how well nonpregnant women feel at the monthly estrogen peak—confident, powerful, creative, physically alert, and strong—and juxtapose this to pregnancy, when estrogen levels soar. Elevated oxytocin and DHEA levels also contribute to a heightened state of awareness.

The Second Trimester

The midpoint of pregnancy is a time of stability. All the basic hormonal and mechanical adjustments have already taken place and now begin to blend with the mother's own efforts to eat, exercise, and rest responsively. Women love this phase; they feel wonderful and look radiant. Around twenty weeks, most mothers feel the baby move for the first time, an event known as quickening. This is an interesting term, connoting awakening and heightened awareness. Some women say they can sense the baby's personality by how it moves, learn about its nature by its rhythms of activity and rest. Most women quite naturally incorporate feelings for the baby into lovemaking with their partner as the dyad becomes a triad. There is no doubt that women in the second trimester have exceptional powers of perception, concentration, and recuperation, all of which enhance sexual expression. Greater physical equilibrium also serves to boost the libido.

Alice, mother of three, puts it this way:

> With each of my pregnancies, I became familiar with my baby a little sooner. The first time, I could barely believe I had a baby in me at all, it was just so overwhelming. Then, I remember an incident with my second: I had the flu and was quite sick, and after a rather violent episode of vomiting I said out loud, "Oh, I hope she's all right." Yes, I had a girl! With the last, though, I felt I knew him right from the start. I would tell people that he was very active, but sweet, and they'd look at me indulgently. It's easy to see now that I was right.

And what about sex with this awareness?

> When it comes to sex, I also felt that I had more ability each time to communicate my knowledge of the baby to my partner. Our deep connection to each other during lovemaking began to include the baby, too, especially with the last one. This was so wonderful—memories I will always treasure. I was with child and the man I love at the same time, and I felt completely fulfilled.

Lesbian mothers report that their experience of alignment in nonpregnant cycles makes possible an even deeper physical empathy in pregnancy that enables both parents to know the baby intimately, even though one partner has no biological link. From Jen: "Sex with Anne when she was pregnant was an ever-so-much enhanced version of what we had known before. I felt very connected to the baby.

Knowing Anne so well, it was easy to differentiate the baby's energy from hers."

Throughout pregnancy, oxytocin levels continue to rise. Oxytocin initiates Braxton-Hicks contractions, which tone the uterus and prepare it for labor. In large amounts, oxytocin has also been shown to cause mood elevation and alleviate depression—perhaps this accounts for the feelings of joy and well-being many women experience at this stage of pregnancy. Take ample amounts of oxytocin, mix with high levels of estrogen, blend with vaginal engorgement, and no wonder many women in their second trimester find themselves sexually insatiable, surprising both themselves and their partners. Jeanine states:

> To be perfectly honest, I masturbated almost every day. It felt very natural to me. Jack was worried that sex would hurt the baby, but our doctor told him to forget his fears. My vagina was so pliable—he could put two or three fingers inside me and I still wanted more, more pressure. I felt like I was opening up for the baby, but when I had orgasms my muscles squeezed so tight Jack said it practically hurt.

Let's take a closer look at men's reactions to sex in pregnancy. If a man feels concern about jeopardizing the pregnancy during the first trimester, his fear may be further compounded by feeling the baby move in the second. The average male believes the vagina to be somewhat delicate, and the idea of deep thrusting close to where a baby is developing makes some men squeamish. But there is more. A surprising number of men struggle with conflicting images of Madonna/Whore, the Mother versus the Lover, unable to blend the two and hence uncertain of how to relate to their pregnant partner sexually. That a woman nurturing new life might also be blatantly lustful and erotic is a powerful merger of two culturally disparate views of femininity. (Witness the stir caused by Demi Moore's infamous pose in *Vanity Fair*: eight months pregnant and wearing nothing but black bra, panties, and spike heels!) Not only for the outright misogynist deeply at odds with his feminine side, but even for the ordinary guy who up to this point has had no idea that such a configuration was possible, there is a strong likelihood of sexual inhibition or shutdown.

What's a woman to do if this occurs? Perhaps her care provider could reassure the father, refer him to a support group or to individual counseling. Deeply ingrained beliefs of this kind are not easy to change, so the situation may not readily improve. For this and many other reasons, women must rely on one another's support, sharing frank discussion along with body-affirming activities like dance or exercise. Although it may seem odd at first, singing with others is also helpful, because it frees the heart and opens the throat. There is a recognized neuromuscular association between the mouth and the vagina: if one is tight, so will the other be.

In many cultures, ritual dance of some sort has been regularly practiced by pregnant women. Contrary to popular belief, belly dancing was not developed to please or seduce men, but rather to support and reinforce the efforts of women in labor. The movements of the dance—rolling hips and the undulating belly—tend naturally to occur during labor in women free of inhibitions. Considering the discomfort and pain of the birth process, a circle of dancing women must have helped remind the mother of how to let go, at the same time echoing her emotional and physical responses in a deeply bonding experience for all. Where, in our institutionalized birthing system, might we find the privacy and support to do the same?

To return to the issue of Mother/Lover role conflict, it is important to add that some women feel this too and may manifest it either by avoiding sex or by wanting to focus exclusively on the baby. Resulting problems may be considerable; disrupted intimacy in a rapidly changing relationship will breed estrangement and mistrust unless lines of communication are kept open. In my practice, I remind women of the sexual nature of birth and use that as a reference point to encourage them to stay open to their partners as much as possible. If the woman is heterosexual, I suggest she experiment with positions such as side-lying or being on top, which will give her more control over the depth of penetration and the rate of thrusting. Labor is, after all, an intensely physical experience; the estimated caloric output of the first birth is equivalent to that of a fifty-mile hike! And it involves the same kind of emotional surrender as spontaneous orgasm.

An important aside here about physical and sexual abuse: more and more women are becoming aware of forgotten or repressed experiences, now that support is available. For many, the emotional vulnerability of pregnancy may trigger recollections for the first time that are doubly difficult to handle if their parents or other relatives are implicated. The accompanying sorrows and fears are apt to interfere with the primary relationship. But wherever possible, it is better to bring these to the surface while pregnant than to have them arise on their own and interfere with labor or mothering. Precisely because pregnancy is such a labile state, I recommend hypnotherapy, which can be especially useful for reactivating and healing the past.

Other psychological barriers to intimacy may involve anxieties about money, role changes, and security. Any woman who finds herself at a sexual impasse while pregnant should make every effort to find assistance.

Here's a relevant account from Mariann:

> I went to a woman's psychotherapy conference while pregnant and took a workshop on sexual abuse. I didn't even know why I was there, really—just for the info, I thought. We went around the room with introductions, and after the first few heart-wrenching accounts, I felt somewhat out of

place. But after a time, I remembered something that happened to me as a child, something I'd completely blocked out. I guess I thought it was no big deal—I was fondled by a conductor on a train when I was twelve—but that day, I relived all of my shame and confusion. I learned that women often tend to minimize these experiences, even though they have a lot of impact. Just being aware of what happened to me shed light on certain aspects of my personality and the way I am with sex. Being pregnant, I felt open enough to make some changes.

No matter what a woman's personal challenges, mid-pregnancy is a fine time for integration, a time to find stability and prepare for the changes ahead.

This, or early in the third trimester, is also an opportune time for a ritual celebration of the pregnancy and forthcoming birth. Increasingly, women in our culture are honored by their loved ones with a special ceremony, something more in depth than the conventional baby shower. In Native American tradition, a Blessingway is performed for every pregnant woman/couple. See the boxed section on page 113 for ideas for a contemporary "Birthingway" celebration.

The Third Trimester

By overview, the first trimester is an initiation into pregnancy; the second, integration and equilibrium; and the third, completion and transition to labor and parenting. Sexuality is often disrupted at this third stage by natural physical discomforts caused by extra weight. Sleep may be sporadic as comfortable positions become harder to find, although lying on the side with pillows between the legs and under the belly can help. Heartburn is commonly caused both by the uterus compressing the stomach and by progesterone softening the esophageal valve so that stomach acids rise upward; thus, a woman may find that the only way she can sleep is propped upright. And she may need to urinate several times nightly, because of increased pressure from the baby against the bladder. None of this is particularly conducive to amour, but the midday rendezvous, or other creative solutions, can help.

Additionally, pelvic cartilage is softened considerably in the third trimester by both progesterone and estrogen, so that ordinary pressure on the pubic bone becomes uncomfortable. Many women long to feel their partners on top of them, or dream of sleeping on their stomach. These longings, combined with the inconvenience of interrupted sleep, promote readiness to give up pregnancy and get on with labor, simultaneously preparing a woman for the challenges of caring for her newborn.

Backache is another major complaint at this time, as the enlarged uterus greatly distends the abdominal muscles and pulls the back out of alignment. Rocking the pelvis on hands and knees, while standing or even while driving, helps tremendously. Of course, pelvic rocking comes naturally with intercourse, as does increased circulation, which can soothe and heal the lower back as well.

Emotionally, these are trying times, with mixed feelings in relationships. Sometimes a woman wants to cling to her partner and hold back time, aware that the baby will soon be out in the world (or in the middle of the bed) and nothing will ever be the same again. Sometimes she wants the privacy just to be with the baby, trying to get to know it as well as she can before it is born, so that sex seems extraneous or more for her partner than for herself. Especially when she is thinking of the challenges ahead and her ongoing need for support, a woman may be demanding, moody, or fearful. Other times, she will feel fully confident, excited by the future and ready to make love to her partner with joy and abandon.

Hormones are at least partially responsible for this spectrum of response, as they are once again on the move, shifting around erratically in preparation for birth. In the last week or so, a drop in progesterone as a precursor to labor often leads to loss of water weight and a feeling of lightness and well-being. Substances called prostaglandins, fatty acids found in the brain, lungs, kidneys, and prostate gland as well as in seminal and menstrual fluids, also increase at term and may be responsible for labor's onset. Or it may be the fetus that is responsible; it too releases prostaglandins as its brain matures. Prostaglandins soften the cervix and cause uterine contractions. Although oxytocin also serves to stimulate uterine activity, it appears less critical in initiating labor and more important in promoting its progress than prostaglandins.

This is why many care providers now encourage intercourse at term, especially if the baby is overdue. Seminal fluid is extremely high in prostaglandins and thus may help trigger labor. (A substitute may be found in evening primrose oil, reputed to have a similar effect when rubbed gently on the cervix.) Sheila Kitzinger, author of *Woman's Experience of Sex* and numerous books on pregnancy, recommends this sexual technique for getting labor going. She advises that a woman make love on her back, well supported by pillows under her hips, her partner kneeling between her legs, her ankles on his shoulders to allow for the deepest penetration. After he ejaculates, she should stay with hips elevated for at least fifteen minutes, so that prostaglandins may be well absorbed by the cervix. Nipple stimulation every ten minutes or so can also help start labor by stimulating the release of oxytocin and subsequent uterine activity. This technique replicates the medical practice of using prostaglandin suppositories to "ripen" the cervix, followed by an intravenous pitocin (synthetic oxytocin) drip to induce contractions. Given the choice, most women would probably choose the non-medical approach, both to avoid the intrusion of technology and to enhance intimacy as labor begins.

Labor and Birth

As labor starts, pregnancy is ending. Many women feel sadness at this, especially if it is to be the last baby or if the pregnancy itself has been especially fulfilling. Others may feel trepidation with the dawning realization that the only way out of labor is through it. Fortunately, women tend to experience a burst of energy at labor's onset, caused by a peak in estrogen and the added effects of oxytocin.

Is childbirth really a sexual event? How can this be, when it's reputed to be so painful? And if birth is sexual in the usual sense, how do women cope in impersonal hospital settings, surrounded by relative strangers?

Let's consider these questions one at a time. Birth as a sexual event—however can we doubt it? After all, it is an intensely physical experience centered in a woman's vagina. In fact, the entire pelvic area is highly stimulated in labor: not just the vagina but the clitoris, rectum, anus, and the supporting tissues and musculature. We can compare the sensations of labor contractions to those of strong menstrual cramps, but with one important difference. Contractions come in waves; they build up steadily instead of taking hold abruptly. Women who have learned to cope with menstrual cramps by relaxing, staying loose and letting go, have a distinct advantage in labor. And here is where the parallels to sexual intercourse begin. Particularly when sex is very passionate and forceful, there may be moments of pain or cramping discomfort with deep thrusting and intense pelvic movement, particularly if the cervix is being hit directly or the uterus is jolted against the intestines. Relaxation, rhythmic breathing, and a change of position help a woman ease through these sensations without losing momentum, as she would if she tightened up or shut down emotionally. Especially with orgasm, the ability to surrender and diffuse sensation throughout the body is critical.

Deep relaxation, surrender, letting go: when midwives are asked to disclose the secret of giving birth with relative ease, these are the words we choose. More than metaphors for coping, these responses are based on physiological imperatives, as we will see in the following sections. We will also look closely at how environment affects the spontaneity of the birth process.

First-Stage Labor

The first stage is the phase of labor when the cervix dilates fully to allow the baby to begin its passage through the vagina and into the world. The cervical opening is ordinarily closed or stretchy only a fingertip's worth; now it will dilate to a circle of approximately ten centimeters in diameter. Over the course of labor, oxytocin intensifies contractions and brings them closer together, which speeds dilation.

In early labor, up to about four centimeters of dilation, contractions may be scarcely noticeable. They may feel more like waves of pelvic warmth "with an edge" than painful cramping. So how about making love during early labor? Considering the link between sex and the release of oxytocin, this is really quite a good idea. A caution, though: most practitioners feel that vaginal penetration should be avoided once the waters have broken, lest infection occur. But generally, intercourse in early labor relaxes the pelvis, gets the hormones pumping, and eases both partners into an intimate and relaxed state conducive to ready progress. Especially if labor is prolonged in the early phase, sex may be just the thing to get it going.

Some women feel like staying just shy of orgasm; others do not. Celine reports, "Just being close with our clothes off, being caressed, helped me relax a lot and take the contractions in stride. I don't know why, but kissing was especially good! Even though my partner eventually came inside me, I felt more like taking it easy than focusing on orgasm."

Kissing and letting go—remember the neuromuscular association between mouth and vagina? In her wonderful book *Spiritual Midwifery*, Ina May Gaskin tells of one couple she directed to kiss in a certain way: the woman with her lips on top, spread out over her partner's. This led to a tangible shift in labor's intensity and very rapid progress. As the classic line from this book reminds us, "The same energy that gets the baby in, gets the baby out."[2]

Couples who do make love in early labor are often thrilled to discover a dimension in lovemaking never before experienced. I have definitely learned my lesson about knocking before entering the labor room, particularly when attending home births. I can think of several times when couples hurriedly pulled their clothes back on or grabbed a blanket, only to have me tell them to go right ahead!

Still, no matter how well a woman has prepared and how eagerly she has anticipated her labor, there may come a time when the going gets rough, as the sensations begin to exceed her expectations. This is the point when preconceptions about what labor will be like, plus ideas about how one should cope and behave, must be swept aside for the real thing. In these moments of reckoning, a woman often finds she must go further in letting go, both physically and emotionally, than she ever has before. It dawns on her that labor is bigger than she is, beyond her experience or control. This can be rather frightening, as it tends to occur fairly early, at just four or five centimeters' dilation. She may feel that she has already tried everything and still cannot handle it. Truth is, she's not going to handle or do it as her ordinary self; she must let herself be transformed to find the way. As you may surmise, this is also a time when many women ask for drugs, particularly if they feel unsupported or exposed.

Imagine yourself in the hospital (not exactly an intimate environment), struggling with labor sensations much stronger than you expected, and painful the second you tense up or break your concentration. The constant stream of medical personnel in and out of your room makes it nearly impossible to let go and relax. You find yourself afraid, wanting to cry out and find relief or move around and change positions, but you just can't; your circumstances are far too inhibiting. Your attendants are sympathetic, but no one is really getting down to your level, looking you in the eye. Though your partner is standing by, she or he also feels afraid and helpless.

Niles Newton, to whom we must be forever grateful for her groundbreaking research on birth, breast-feeding, and sexuality, investigated the importance of environmental factors on the birth of mice. She found that births were longer and more difficult when mice were placed in unfamiliar surroundings, could not smell or see what they were used to, were moved repeatedly during labor, or were placed in clear (as opposed to opaque) cages. Opposite factors of familiar surroundings, privacy, and stability contributed to spontaneous, easy deliveries.[3]

It was Grantly Dick-Read, author of *Childbirth Without Fear*, who first revealed how fear or tension can cause pain and lack of progress in labor. Starting with a review of basic physiology, he explained that the uterus is composed of several muscular layers: an outer layer featuring longitudinal fibers and an inner layer with circular fibers. In the absence of fear or tension, oxytocin causes the long fibers not only to contract but to retract and become shorter, pulling on inner fibers encircling the cervix and causing dilation. But when a woman is frightened or tense, elevated adrenaline levels shunt blood away from the uterus and cause the circular fibers to become rigid. The two muscle layers then work against each other, and pain results.[4] Similarly, if you are tense or frightened during intercourse, you are not likely to experience orgasm.

How to avoid all this? Picture yourself in a darkened room with just your partner, the two of you in bed relaxing in each other's arms, your midwife or doctor sitting quietly in the corner, coming over now and then to check the baby and offer encouragement, then perhaps retiring to an adjacent area so your privacy is complete. You still have to deal with the pain, both the physical intensity and the psychological shock of "it's not what I expected," but you can speak freely to your partner, you can cry, laugh, shout, or do whatever else suits you as you work together; it is your experience.

A major problem with hospital birth is increasingly routine interventions in otherwise normal labor. Once the decision is made for one such intervention, others are likely to follow. For example, when pitocin is used to speed up labor (whether because of hospital guidelines for progress or for the convenience of the obstetrician), contractions often become so unnaturally strong and painful that the mother requires pain relief. These contractions may also stress the baby, because when the uterus is forced beyond its capacity and does not relax fully between contractions, circulation is impaired and the baby receives less oxygen through the umbilical cord. If fetal distress intensifies, the probable conclusion is Cesarean birth.

Consider that one in five births in the United States today is by Cesarean section; in some hospitals, the rate is as many as one in three. This is shocking but not really surprising, so deeply do we fear the mystery of women's bodies and so strongly do we venerate control. Some women even request Cesarean birth for much the same reasons; it seems less threatening and easier to handle than vaginal birth. Little do they know that Cesarean section is major abdominal surgery, nor are they told how difficult recovery can be when one must deal with postoperative pain and tend a baby, establish breast-feeding, suffer sleep deprivation, and cope with the sweeping physiological and emotional changes of the postpartum period.

Old medical texts teach that less than 5 percent of births involve complications. Our 20 to 30 percent Cesarean rate has mostly iatrogenic causes—that is, those generated by technology, procedure, or practitioner. The fact that our malpractice compensation system does not discriminate between acts of fate and genuine negligence has forced medical practice to be increasingly defensive, based more on conservative protocol than on what the data show. Under fear of lawsuit, every possible test and procedure will be run, no matter how painful or irrelevant to the mother's condition. Add to this our culturally inculcated expectation of perfection, and the high rate of Cesarean birth becomes even more understandable. Nevertheless, the fact remains that birth is a mystery, one that can never be fully circumscribed by technology. Even in the most carefully monitored situations, hemorrhages occur unexpectedly, babies get stuck at the shoulder, cord accidents happen at the last minute, babies and mothers die. The bottom line is that here in the United States, in spite of all our intervention, we have a higher perinatal mortality rate than most countries where birth occurs spontaneously and is commonly attended at home. Thus, women (and their supporters) must make every effort to see beyond propaganda and marketing to make truly informed decisions regarding the birth attendant and place of birth.

Whatever your environment, once you make the shift to active labor—with contractions long and strong, coming about every five minutes—neurohormones called endorphins begin to enter your bloodstream. These are commonly released with intense physical activity and are responsible for the surge of strength, power and well-being known as a "second wind" or "runner's high." Once her endorphins have kicked in, a woman may actually enjoy labor or may even find it an ecstatic experience. I have many times told the story of one of my clients who was crying and desperate in early labor, only to be smiling and dancing around the room at nine centimeters' dilation. Not every woman maintains an external focus so far into labor; it depends on how quickly her labor is progressing and how strong contractions are. Many women turn inward as they approach full dilation, eyes closed between contractions and peacefully out of body. Still, there is always the exception, like the woman who laughed, chatted, and ate fried chicken until she was ready to push!

Endorphins are, by the way, also released with intercourse and lead to the exquisite feeling known as afterglow. However, if anesthetics or analgesics are used during labor, stress perception will be minimal and endorphin release may not occur. Although pain may be nearly obliterated by medication, so too will the ecstatic, transcendent feelings many women report in giving birth naturally.

What comes next in the birth process? Even women who have never been pregnant have heard of the transition phase of labor, reputed to be the most difficult of all. Not every woman experiences transition, but for those who do, it occurs somewhere between seven to ten centimeters' dilation. Physically, the cervix continues to dilate even as the baby descends through it and pushes onto the pelvic floor. This leads to mixed, conflicting messages of "relax, stay open, surrender," and "push, bear down, get busy!" Just when a woman feels she has finally made her peace with letting go, she suddenly feels compelled to do something, to act. Her emotions swing wildly; she may swear at her partner or birth attendants. Hormonally, ongoing rushes of oxytocin are interspersed with surges of adrenaline.

How can these purportedly conflicting hormones work in concert? According to birth physiology expert Michel Odent, there comes a time in labor, generally at the point dilation gives way to bearing down, when adrenaline is both physiologic and positive in effect. He explains that there are actually two different types of uterine receptors for adrenaline: beta-inhibitory and alpha-initiatory. Adrenaline is also a

precursor to prostaglandin release—bringing to mind the characteristic burst of energy just before labor starts—and increased
prostaglandin levels are thought to be responsible for the bearing-down
reflex. Tying human physiology to animal behavior in the wild, Odent
notes that if threatened in early labor, a mother usually waits until she
can safely give birth, but if labor is well advanced or happening
quickly, it is to her advantage to give birth as soon as possible.[5]

Odent notes that the natural release of adrenaline at this stage may
be accompanied by surges of fear or anxiety. But is adrenaline a
precursor to these emotions, or is it the other way around? In either
case, at least if a woman experiences panic, she can feel comforted in
knowing it is normal. She may even have mortal fear and feel as
though she must fight for survival. She may well cry out or scream.
This is in direct contrast to what is taught in most childbirth preparation classes, that women should make only low-pitched sounds lest
they tighten up, and they should make the transition to second-stage
labor as calmly as possible. On the contrary, women left to their own
devices often scream or roar as they enter second stage, sometimes
leaping to their feet or into a crouch with superhuman strength. These
same women later revel in the power of this moment. "Those sounds,"
one recalled, "where were they coming from? Some deep part of me
that had never been touched before. They rang in my ears—raw, clear,
and unbelievably strong." "I felt so primal," said another, "like some
sort of tigress, a jungle queen." For many, this is one of the most sexual
moments in giving birth, one that can transform a previously shy or
inhibited woman into a powerfully assertive lover.

Second-Stage Labor

To backtrack a bit, we must clarify that although second-stage labor
commences with full dilation, some women do not experience the
adrenaline surge and urge to push for some time after, especially if the
baby is still fairly high in the pelvis. Sometimes, if labor has been long

or hard thus far, women even sleep or nap as the uterus rests, then wake with clear urges to push. As bearing-down signals get stronger, pressure begins to build in the vagina. What is this sensation like? Imagine something the size of a grapefruit (the baby's head) pressing hard on all the sensitive areas deep inside you, combined with a downward squeezing urge something like moving your bowels but ten times stronger—a whole-body urge turning you inside out—and you have some idea of the sensory magnitude as delivery approaches. No wonder we need a burst of adrenaline to help us through! Physiologically, the uterus has stretched and thinned in the lower segment, while the long fibers have retracted to form a strong mass at the top that pushes the baby downward. And it is primarily the uterus that pushes the baby out, not the mother, although her ability to cooperate with her body makes a difference in the ease of progress. Second stage can consist of twenty minutes of urges so overwhelming that you can scarcely catch your breath, or it may last several hours with urges of varying length and intensity, sometimes so light you can breathe right through them.

Once again, however, we find medical management at odds with basic physiology; labor and delivery staff seem determined in nearly every case to get the baby out as soon as possible. Women are told to draw their legs back forcibly, hold a breath as long as possible, and push their guts out with every contraction. This is rather like trying to force orgasm, riding over the rhythm instead of with it. To put it another way, under which circumstances might you find it easier to have an orgasm: with someone barking orders at you every step of the way, or when free to surrender to your body and let it take you? Most probably, aggressive management of second stage is a remnant of old notions that it is dangerous for both mother and baby to let the fetal head "pound the perineum." It may also signify an inculcated fear of the vagina as a "dangerous" place. In reality, forced, insensitive pushing is apt to cause damage to vaginal tissues, at the same time depriving the baby of oxygen. As demonstrated by Roberto Caldeyro-Barcia, unnaturally long periods of maternal breath-holding can lead to fetal acidosis and distress.[6] Author Sheila Kitzinger goes so far as to say that medicine has imposed a male-ejaculation model on the pushing process, for which the variable-intensity, multiple-orgasm female model is imminently more suitable.[7]

When a woman in second stage is unfettered by outside direction, she will, in fact, breathe very much as she would during sexual excitation and orgasm: up to three times more rapidly than usual, with periods of breath-holding punctuated by gasps, groans, or cries. Women allowed to push their babies out spontaneously do describe delivery in sexual terms, speaking of tremendous release, ecstatic rushes of emotion, and overwhelming happiness. I have observed that if women are controlled by others while pushing, they are somewhat inhibited at first with their babies.

For me, the ecstasy of second stage occurred when my uterus and I were working as one, beyond signal and response. In this mode, a woman can literally deliver her own baby, sensing exactly when she can take more stretch and when to ease up, gently breathing her baby out. I had been given a huge episiotomy (a cut to enlarge the birth canal) with my first birth, so I was determined not to tear with the second. I really tuned in during pushing—just closed my eyes and did it all from the inside. I could feel everything, the precise contours of my daughter's head as I eased it out, even her little shoulders and body as she whooshed and squiggled through. It was absolutely the most exquisite thing I have ever felt in my life. Later, my midwives said they wished they had videotaped the birth, because it was so perfectly controlled. But for me, control had nothing to do with it, as I wasn't holding back. Beyond attunement, there was union—perfect union.

There has been some important research done regarding vaginal stimulation in labor and subsequent bonding behaviors. Vaginal stimulation has been shown to be an important determinant of bonding in

sheep.[8] When nonpregnant ewes primed with estrogen and progesterone were vaginally stimulated (by vibrator), they responded to
newborn lambs with a full range of bonding behaviors. With the same
stimulation, ewes that had recently delivered and had already bonded
to their own lambs stopped rejective behavior toward foreign lambs
and accepted them as their own. Further, Krehbiel and co-workers
found that giving peridural (pelvic floor) anesthetic to birthing ewes,
particularly if given early, severely altered normal maternal behavior;
seven of the eight first-time mothers failed to show any bonding
response in the first half hour. Ewes that had given birth previously
responded less dramatically but still showed some effects.[9] Perhaps the
choice of epidural anesthesia, which numbs to a greater extent than
does peridural, is not so benign as we have thought. I have noticed that
once an epidural is administered, a woman becomes more a spectator
of her birth than a participant. She is often at a loss as to what to do
with her newborn, whereas the unmedicated mother usually responds
to her baby passionately, with fiercely protective instincts.

This raises yet another issue, that of vaginal tearing with delivery.
Isn't it better to have an episiotomy, rather than being stretched out or
torn? And if an episiotomy is going to be necessary, then mustn't the
area be numbed in advance anyway?

Here we have one of the biggest lies perpetuated by modern obstetrics: that the human vagina is somehow inadequate to the task of
delivery and must be surgically enhanced to accomplish it. Most
women don't realize that the vagina's surface is covered with ruggae,
accordion-like folds of tissue that expand naturally with the hormonal
effects of pregnancy. When a woman is relaxed and centered at
delivery, not rushed but well supported, she will generally give birth
without a scratch, or with abrasions so minor they require no treatment. And despite beliefs to the contrary, episiotomies do not heal
better than tears: if a tear does require stitches, its irregular edges actu-

ally mesh together better and close more quickly than the clean-edged episiotomy wound. Finally, it is much easier to regain sexual pleasure and muscle responsiveness after repair of a tear than an episiotomy. Tears frequently skim the surface, but in doing an episiotomy one is obliged to cut deeply through muscle. The result is a wall of scar tissue, both inflexible and numb to sensation.

But what about vaginal snugness after birth? How can an area that has been stretched so dramatically ever regain its former tone? Isn't that what the "husband's knot" is for? What disgusting terminology! And what's worse, this excessively tight stitch at the base of the vaginal opening does little more than cause pain and distress with intercourse. Pleasurable friction is found not at the opening anyway, but from muscles immediately inside the vagina, which extend upward several inches or so. Although it is possible to create a tight vaginal opening with surgical repair, scarred areas inside will be rigid, surrounding muscles flaccid, and the entire area dysfunctional for many months. But when the vagina is intact after birth, the muscles continue to respond as a unit. Keep in mind that when a woman is fully aroused, she naturally tightens at the vaginal opening and just inside, while the back portion of the canal balloons several inches longer and wider — nature's design to allow seminal fluid to pool around the cervix. In general, the woman who has given birth naturally and has retoned her vaginal muscles postpartum will be a more responsive and pleasurable partner than one with deep-tissue trauma and repair (at least until healing occurs, which can take a long time).

In the 1950s, when the "husband's knot" became a standard part of repair technique, women were not taught pelvic floor exercises (see Chapter 5), and few explored their own musculature for fear of hurting themselves or doing something "dirty." Sexual mores were based on male gratification; little was known or understood about female sexual response. Times have changed; women are more embodied now, and most have no qualms about putting their fingers inside the vagina to help them locate and tone the muscles there. Women who are in touch with themselves like this and who have prepared to give birth without an episiotomy often feel violated and emotionally traumatized if they get one anyhow. As one woman, Jan, said of her first birth, "I felt I was doing a good job, easing my baby out nicely, when suddenly and for no apparent reason my doctor changed his mind and cut me. I felt defeated, like, 'Oh . . . well, okay, I give up . . . guess I'm not good enough.' I lost all feeling, and he took control."

I have assisted more than three hundred births and have only had to perform episiotomy five times, each because of last-minute fetal distress necessitating immediate delivery. Seldom do women in my practice tear, and if they do, the tear is usually minor and requires no stitches. This is no miracle; it's simply a matter of helping women tune into their sensations, engaging them in sensitive breathing, using hot compresses and perineal massage to stimulate circulation and relaxation, reminding them to take it slowly.

Delivery

At the final moment of crowning, when the widest part of the baby's head stretches the vaginal opening to its maximum, some women love either to look in a mirror or to reach down and touch their little one for the first time. Sometimes this brings a tremendous flood of emotion, and the baby is born in an orgasm of delivery. Most women describe the moment of delivery as the high point of their lives, a physical and emotional pinnacle. All the waiting and wondering, all hopes and fears are finally unleashed and allowed to rush forward as the baby swooshes out and utters its first cry.

If she feels like it, the mother can reach down and lift the baby up when it is still partly inside her—something she will never forget. The baby is wet, warm, incredibly fragile yet surprisingly strong. It smells sweetly of birth. She touches its little hands and feet and then finds herself falling into its eyes, seeing the faces of relatives and ancestors, feeling past and future unite. Birth is a stunning victory for a woman, especially when she has retained her power and knows she has given it her all.

Birth Is a Blood Mystery

◉

The real truth is that birth is a mystery, one by which we grow and learn exponentially as compared to ordinary life lessons. Here is a tale of our heritage as birthing women.

* * *

Once, women walked the world in beauty and confidence. They were revered and kept safe by their communities. When such a woman came to her time to give birth, she had already seen the births of siblings or other relatives, or had assisted her close women friends. She had no question of her body's worth and power, no fear of rape or abuse. Her menarche had been cause for great celebration; she was guided through this rite of passage with ritual and song—and it was deeply joyous! Now she would explore the unknown once again, but within the container of meaning given by her culture, supported by a circle of women of all ages, and guided by the midwives.

She was nourished well as labor began, bathed and adorned. As her pains became stronger, she began her journey to the birth hut. Along her way were a series of upright poles she could use for support; she moved to the next only when labor dramatically intensified, so that by the time she reached the birth hut she was nearly ready. There her circle of supporters surrounded her more closely, dancing sensually, chanting and smiling, touching her as needed. The passion of birth took her completely, and she surrendered to its power. As she did so, pain became interspersed with ecstasy, and she sank into blissful rest between each contraction, her spirit traveling far and wide. Soon she felt urges to push and became more upright, held and encouraged, gentle hands brushing her hair back from her forehead. She had never felt so open, so boundless and vulnerable, yet so strong. Her baby moving down inside her brought new sensations, so much intensity, yet still she could clearly feel its exquisite form. She gave way completely, panting and surging, and her baby glided out into the world onto the bed of soft grass beneath her. What wonder, what beauty, what joy! She reached down to touch and slowly took the baby up with her hands and into her arms. Her placenta was soon birthed, handled carefully that its ritual and healing powers might be preserved.

In the weeks that followed, she and her partner were fed and cared for by the women elders. Each day, and for long periods of time, she was attended by these women, who saw to her per-sonal needs, chatted with her about community affairs, and instructed her in her new role. A fire was kept burning to keep her living space warm enough for her to be without clothes, so she might readily heal and breast-feed with ease. After a period of six weeks, she and her baby were officially welcomed by the community. When her best friend gave birth a year later, she was at her side with confidence and encouragement.

* * *

In the next chapter, we will explore the tender and tempestuous postpartum period and look at how sexual identity and expression are affected and transformed by the presence of a newborn.

The Birthingway

The Birthingway, which has its roots in Native American tradition, is a rite to prepare the mother-to-be to surrender to the mysteries of labor and birth. It is a powerful ceremony honoring the pregnant woman's strength and beauty as life-bringer.

Birth rituals are intended to help parents accept a new person into their midst, but they also strengthen the ties that bind us together in community. In the Sudan, each pregnant woman is honored in a ceremony similar to Native American tradition. Her hair is hennaed, braided, and scented, she wears a special bracelet and leather thong around her waist for protection, and she lies on a ceremonial mat of palm leaf stems. Her relatives then gather around to rub her belly with handfuls of millet porridge—vitamin-rich and symbolic of regeneration. In the Mansi tradition, women assist the expectant mother by ritual preparation of birch bark cradles, special coverlets of swan skin, and pillows of deer fur twice the size of the mother's hand; once these are ready, they begin work on a reed mattress on which the new mother will sit and sleep for a certain number of days following her child's birth. Regardless of cultural specifics, the common purpose of prenatal ceremony is to empower the mother as her time draws near and to replace fear with affirmations of her sacredness as the gateway for new life.

Birthingways of today are basically gatherings of the mother's closest women friends and relatives, who bring gifts to honor her and her baby. They may wish to create ritual space by smudging with sage or cedar, or may simply choose to sit in a circle and talk, sharing words of wisdom regarding the challenges of motherhood, or perhaps a favorite anecdote regarding birth or child rearing. The mother's hair may then be combed and adorned with feathers, ribbons, and shells, her crown bedecked with flowers. Some mothers save these ornaments and use them to make mobiles to hang above the crib. Traditionally, the mother's feet are bathed in herbal teas and rubbed dry with cornmeal (once known as the "Santo Domingo" foot rub, this feels heavenly). Bathing and rubbing the mother's feet signifies the wish that she will successfully walk the holy path of labor and birth.

All in the circle may then unite by lightly looping a length of red yarn around their wrists one at a time, to symbolize the umbilical cord connection each had to her own mother. A bowl with red-stained eggs (dyed in beet juice and traditional at Birthingways) can then be passed around the circle, and each woman in turn may speak three blessings: one for the mother, one for the baby, and one for the global community of women. The mother may also be given poetry and song as gifts. Sometimes she is presented with a bundle or pouch of sacred objects.

When it is time to open the circle, the red yarn is cut so that each woman can keep a bracelet around her wrist to hold the mother in her thoughts until she has had her baby. The eggs blessed in the circle are usually buried outside in a special place, where the placenta might later be buried with a tree or rosebush planted above it. (Women who birth in hospital can, by the way, request that their placenta be given to them to take home.)

Most important in creating these rites is that we stay flexible, letting the personality of the prospective mother be the basis for our design. A simple format involves a gathering for the purpose of making a birth garment for her to wear during her labor, such as an oversized T-shirt decorated with fabric pens, stitchery, sequins, etc. As they make the garment, the women can sing or tell stories about birth. At the same time, they may also wish to make a small garment for the baby. Or they could gather to make a quilt, each of them creating their own squares in advance, then assembling them together.

Another simple gesture is the Apache tradition of presenting the mother with a basket cornucopia full of fruits, candy, nuts, and money to symbolize abundance in the four life stages of infancy, childhood, adulthood, and old age.

Whatever form it takes, the ceremony is always followed by feasting and levity. At this point, men may also join the party. This is not to say the father can't have his own ritual celebration— perhaps earlier, while the mother was circling with the women, his male friends and relations might have taken him aside to offer their own anecdotes and words of wisdom regarding parental responsibilities. However, particularly since birth takes place in the mother's body, it is crucial that the Birthingway be centered on her. As it concludes, she should feel blessed by her loved ones and infused with love and courage.

Reprinted from *The Women's Wheel of Life: Thirteen Archetypes of Woman at Her Fullest Power,* by Elizabeth Davis and Carol Leonard

Sex after the Baby Comes

The postpartum period is defined as a minimum of six weeks and a maximum of three years after giving birth. This is undoubtedly one of the sweetest and most challenging times of a woman's life. It has wisely been said that the exhilaration of pregnancy and birth are but preparation for the grueling adjustments to be made postpartum. I often tell women that the first six weeks of caring for a newborn is the hardest work they will ever do. The changes involved in adding another member to the family are far from minor, and the stress of it all may well lead a woman (and her partner) to wonder whether there is sex after birth.

The Recovery Process

With a little patience and creativity, sex usually comes back better than ever, even though modifications are called for at first. To truly understand sexuality during this phase, we must look at the physical process of recovery as well as that of lactation.

In the first few moments following delivery, fresh spurts of oxytocin are released to contract the uterus and shear off the placenta. As the baby is put to the breast, nipple stimulation triggers additional oxytocin, which shrinks the uterus down to the size of a grapefruit. Over the next ten days or so, continued release of oxytocin will contract the uterus back to its pre-pregnant size.

When a woman breast-feeds, oxytocin levels rise even higher according to the frequency of nursing, which in the first few weeks may occur as often as every hour or two. The extra boost serves to contract and tone the upper vaginal area (or vault), a process that takes place much more slowly in women who bottle-feed.

Milk production is initiated in part by the hormone prolactin, which is released when estrogen and progesterone levels drop with delivery. Continued milk production depends on stimulation of the breasts—the more the baby sucks, the more milk the mother will produce, as long as she has adequate rest, food, and drink. Let-down of milk with each nursing is triggered by oxytocin via nipple stimulation. Oxytocin also increases blood flow to the breasts, causing them to radiate heat so the baby is literally bathed in warmth.

What does let-down feel like? For most women, it's very pleasurable. It begins with tingling sensations in the breasts, followed by tightening as they fill, then strong physical urges for release. We have, I think, a ready correlation here to what men experience with arousal. There is an imperative need to be partnered that accompanies let-down: a mother experiencing it wants her baby now.

It seems obvious that breast-feeding is a sexual experience. Sometimes, uterine and vaginal contractions caused by oxytocin even lead to orgasm. Unless a woman has deep inhibitions, breast-feeding is at the very least physically fulfilling, with surges of warmth and well-being that encompass body and soul. And the experience is mutual: the baby responds with love and desire, its little hands stroke the breast, its toes curl rhythmically, its body presses forward (as it gets older). Just as making love bonds emotionally healthy adults together, so does breast-feeding bond mother and child. In fact, suckling at the breast has been shown to trigger the release of oxytocin in the newborn, which not only helps stabilize its mood but facilitates digestion. We are little accustomed to thinking of babies as having sexual needs, but to a certain extent, they do. Close to our most basic definition of sexual desire is the physical and emotional urge for intimacy that is with us from birth.

Niles Newton and Charlotte Modahl found that mood changes occurring with intercourse and orgasm are very much like those that accompany breast-feeding. Women who bottle-feed their babies have been shown to have higher levels of anxiety, stress, depression, and guilt than mothers who breast-feed.[1] According to the research of E. B. Thoman and colleagues, lactating women show a suppression of adrenaline release (and the accompanying neurological activity) in response to trauma.[2] The release of oxytocin through breast-feeding appears to be a biological perk to help women buffer stress and make it through the physical challenges of this phase, such as sleep deprivation, hormonally based moodiness, and sweeping physiological adjustments.

Postpartum adjustment is indeed more than a matter of restoring pelvic anatomy and establishing breast-feeding. Remember the many physiological changes of pregnancy mentioned in the Chapter 4: elevated blood volume, increased thyroid and kidney function, decreases in vascular tension, changes in digestion, and so on. In the first few weeks postpartum, all these shift back to pre-pregnant norms. But this is hardly a smooth, even process of change—it is fitful and erratic. Hormones ebb, flow, and only gradually readjust. The resulting hot flashes and cold spells, night sweats, and mood swings make this a biologically and emotionally charged period for women and their families (quite similar to menopause).

Emotional Change and Adjustment

Distinguishing biologically induced mood swings postpartum from those based on more serious psychological problems can be something of a challenge in this culture. That we treat the new mother as though nothing in her life has changed, expecting her to be back on her feet and in charge of her affairs in a matter of days, is truly the height of denial. In nearly every society but our own, continuous support is provided to all new mothers during their "lying-in" period; their only obligation is to stay in bed and focus on themselves and the baby. Sometimes this lasts six weeks, sometimes only ten days, but in any case, mothering the mother leads her to bond more deeply with her baby and recover more completely. The better she feels, the more easily she will integrate her new role and begin to distinguish the needs of her child from her own. Good care frees her to develop as an individual; it gives her a healthy foundation on which to base her social interactions, present and future. Her child reaps the benefits of security and respect for its own processes of growth. Care of new mothers assures survival of the species, but more than that, it positively affects quality of life for all of us.

Postpartum customs of Native American and Indonesian cultures specifically involve the use of heat. It is understood that new mothers are still open from the birth and are thus physically vulnerable, susceptible to chill and loss of energy. Frequently, a fire is built near or even under the mother's bed so she may nurse spontaneously, remain unclothed, and feel comfortable and at ease. Far from the numbing isolation mothers commonly experience in our society, women of these cultures are surrounded by female peers and extended family who feed and counsel them, laugh with them, and marvel at the miracle of their newborn child. In the Philippines, the new mother is believed to be in such a state of grace that should she die in the first forty days postpartum, her soul automatically goes to heaven.

When a woman is not well cared for at this time, there are complex, often long-term effects on her body, personality, and sexuality. Although oxytocin has the ability to buffer stress, it definitely has its limits. If a woman is forced out of bed or back to work too soon, overproduction of adrenaline will derail her recovery. As Newton observes, "Oxytocin reflexes can be severely inhibited by environmental disturbances, emotional upset or pain."[3] Thus the "Amazon concept" of postpartum recovery can be nothing but myth: women never did give birth in the bush and jump immediately back on their horses, unless their survival depended on it. To put it another way: our scandalously high incidence of postpartum depression here in the United States has frustrated biological needs at its root. Without sufficient rest, postpartum recovery is grueling and prolonged. And sex is on the far back burner.

There are other factors, too. The same cultural ideology that deems it appropriate to abandon the new mother further challenges her changing identity. In assuming her new role, she is bound to experience loss, some of it painful. Single friends may abandon her, finding it impossible to relate to what she is experiencing. Her primary relationship has already been altered; now it may become somewhat strained. She herself is inextricably changed; old routines and ways of handling the most basic tasks no longer work. Privacy seems a thing of the past, at least for the time being. If she takes maternity leave, she may experience a loss of income and concomitant change in her standard of living. And finally, what should be at most a temporary loss of energy and resourcefulness may seem all but permanent to her unless she receives assistance. Chronic fatigue—really very common postpartum—may link to other losses and lead to clinical depression. New mothers are fragile, vulnerable, impressionable, and still quite sensitive from giving birth. Well-meaning but misguided advice sinks deep; criticism is not easily forgotten.

More than anything else, giving birth makes clear that control in life is just an illusion. Ideally, a woman's experience of making this discovery is positive, even exhilarating; if not, her self-esteem may be negatively affected. This can compound depression. One of my most critical tasks in caring for clients postpartum is to help them debrief their birth experience. Women sometimes express anxiety about their performance in labor as early as day three, and they may call again in tearful panic over the next few weeks for more discussion, more reassurance. This is particularly true if the birth has been difficult or the outcome somehow disappointing. Certainly the course of acceptance will be rocky if there are problems with the baby's health or physical condition. But a woman can have a perfectly lovely and healthy baby and still be devastated by her experience of the birth. Until very recently, women were denied the right to grieve their birth disappointments; as my mother was told when she complained to her doctor about the indignities she suffered at the hands of hospital staff, "If the cake is good, eat it!" She told me this just days after my own traumatic first delivery, and it remains one of the fateful moments in my life when I said to myself, "No, that is not enough, I am worth more than that, women are worth more than that!"

Yet another aspect of a mother's recovery has to do with how deeply she has bonded to her baby. Much research has been done in this area, most of it showing damaging effects if mother and baby are separated for more than moments during the first few hours, especially immediately after birth. Animals thus separated respond in classic, predictable ways: the newborn will bond with whatever is available—even another species, or something mechanical—and the mother will reject her young when later reintroduced. This is powerful genetic programming meant to ensure survival, and when it is disrupted in the human sphere a woman feels rather like Humpty Dumpty: who can put the pieces back together again? And if the mother stays in the hospital for more than a few hours, bonding may be further disrupted by nurses who feel obliged (or may choose) to begin caring for the baby: dressing it, changing its diaper, comforting it in her presence. All these are critical tasks the mother needs to handle herself, that she may awaken her natural instincts and develop her own foundation for caregiving.

It is both curious and disappointing that one of our leading feminist thinkers, Gloria Steinem, traces the problem of damaged self-esteem no further back than the early years. She acknowledges that "as infants and small children, we cannot possibly earn our welcome in this world," but she fails to link this to our experience at birth.[4] She stresses the importance of "honoring the wisdom of the body," yet she seems unaware of how deeply this wisdom can be violated by a traumatic birth experience. If birth is perceived as negative and/or bonding is impaired, a chain reaction of missed communication between mother and baby may make efforts to develop the relationship frustrating and exceedingly difficult.

Breast-feeding provides an important way to reestablish bonds that have been broken by difficult birth. Counseling is increasingly available for women who need help with this. And in spite of the crucial importance of bonding at birth, we human females are distinct from other mammals in that we have the intelligence and intent to deliberately re-create our bonds with our young. This is far from easy, but it can be done.

How does this affect postpartum sexuality? At the most basic level, the key to sexual fulfillment in this phase has to do with the mother's self-acceptance and integration. She must recognize her new role, work out her birth experience, acknowledge her changed identity, and deepen her attachment to her baby. If she is able to do all this, she will generally return to her intimate relationship with enthusiasm. There are a few practical concerns regarding sex at this time, but ultimately, sex postpartum is not about timing and technique any more than it is at any other phase of a woman's life. The reason many guidebooks take this focus is that dealing with the underlying issues is daunting, to say the least. But if the only advice we can offer a new mother concerned about her sex life is to make love in the afternoon when the baby sleeps, she is apt to feel that even her sexuality has been pared down to practicality—that it, too, was lost when she gave birth.

There is ample evidence that a good bond between mother and baby makes for better sex. Masters and Johnson found that breast-feeding women had a higher level of sexual interest than bottle-feeding mothers. As a group, they sought as rapid a return as possible to sexual activity with their partners.[5]

But the data are contradictory. Other studies show a marked decline in sexual interest among breast-feeding mothers. This is attributed to the hormone prolactin, which is known to diminish sex drive. However, oxytocin can counteract the effects of prolactin to some extent.

Is there any way to increase the level of oxytocin in our bodies? Studies show that the amount of oxytocin in the systems of breast-feeding women is not at all constant, as one might suspect, but varies dramatically. Mothers who nursed for long stretches tended to have the highest levels overall and also to experience spikes from time to time.[6] High oxytocin levels are associated with increased interest in making love. And we already know that sexual activity itself increases oxytocin.

Yet another substance, a neurotransmitter known as dopamine, tends to modify the effects of prolactin. Dopamine is the "feel-good" hormone associated with desire; it causes us to perceive and pursue pleasure. Sexual activity increases our levels of dopamine.

What does all this mean? The data suggest that although prolactin has a subduing effect on sex drive, women may be able to counteract this both by nursing their babies on demand and by making love. In other words, sex itself may be a remedy for sexual disinterest. You may have already found this to be true empirically: if you have ever gone for long periods without sex, you probably got quite comfortable living without it, but once you resumed sexual activity, you couldn't wait for the next encounter. Perhaps while breast-feeding we must make an effort to have sex in order to keep this cycle going, especially since prolactin will continue to intervene until weaning has occurred.

Practicalities of Postpartum Sex

◎

Now we are ready to discuss the more concrete details of postpartum sexuality. Especially at first, women are greatly concerned about their internal healing and potential vulnerability during lovemaking, particularly if they have had stitches.

Fear is often triggered by either pain or stiffness at the site of injury. Physicians commonly have women return for a checkup at six weeks postpartum to assess the healing of the perineum and make recommendations for contraception, as appropriate. But most women are told little or nothing about how to care for the perineum in the interim, or how to watch for warning signals of infection like swelling or inflammation. Pain is an important signal of problems, too, but it may go unnoticed if a woman is taking painkillers during the first few days, the most critical time for healing.

I suggest that women use ice packs for twenty-four hours to reduce swelling, then switch to sitz baths several times daily using hot water with selected herbs. Nothing speeds healing faster than heat, and soaking is far superior to topical application as it more deeply stimulates circulation. Fresh ginger is a good addition to the solution; it helps relieve the itching that often occurs as stitches dissolve and the skin heals.

Here is how I recommend women take a sitz bath: Grate a three-to-four-inch root into a large pot of water, simmer twenty minutes, strain, and divide into two portions. Save one for later in the day, and dilute the first with water in a sitz bath unit (a special plastic tub that fits directly over the toilet seat, available at most pharmacies). After soaking for twenty minutes, thoroughly dry the perineum and expose to air or sunlight for another ten minutes before putting on a fresh pad (or use a hair dryer to speed the process). If the perineum feels at all sticky, you can use aloe vera gel to dry and soothe the tissues. Avoid vitamin E or other oil-based ointments until the skin is healed over, as these tend to keep edges from closing.

Despite the six-week ban on sex, some women go ahead and make love anyway before returning to their practitioner for permission. Sometimes this is fine; sometimes the experience is so fraught with anxiety and discomfort that it is both worrisome and disappointing. Why the time limit at all? Ordinarily, it takes ten days for the uterus to return to normal size and the cervix to close securely. Sex during this time can cause bleeding beyond normal postpartum amounts. There may also be some risk of uterine infection, although this has never been adequately documented. Stitches are a major contraindication to sex in the first few weeks; they take a week or so to dissolve and at least two more to heal. Any woman who has had stitches should really be checked before having sex, even if it means scheduling an appointment earlier than her practitioner expects or recommends.

Most women are anxious about sex after giving birth. Preliminary self-massage can help, particularly in areas with scar tissue. The wall-like ridge characteristic of episiotomy can be softened and relaxed with thumb or finger pressure, using a little oil (just make sure to wash your hands before handling the baby or breast-feeding). When scarring is extensive, evening primrose oil (found in health-food stores) may significantly help to reduce it. Due to decreased estrogen postpartum, vaginal lubrication may also pose a problem during sex. Water-based lubricating jelly is best for intercourse, as excess oil can clog delicate vaginal tissues and glands.

Estrogen production and the return of the monthly cycle will occur spontaneously if a mother stops breast-feeding or may gradually resume as she introduces solid foods and the baby nurses less often. There are exceptions, though. Some women nurse their babies (or even toddlers) just once or twice a day and still do not resume their normal cycle. Others may nurse exclusively and have milk in abundance, yet start menstruating as early as six weeks postpartum. The reasons for this discrepancy are uncertain. A number of my clients have observed that sexual activity in the first two weeks postpartum seemed to cause them to start menstruating within the next month. No harm in this; certainly, a woman's sex life will benefit. But babies tend to be fussier when their mothers are menstruating, and PMS can be especially trying if combined with sleep deprivation and fatigue.

If adequately repaired and cared for, the perineum should be fully healed at six weeks no matter how extensive the damage. I recently saw a woman (not my client) who was experiencing pain and bleeding with intercourse seven months after perineal repair! She had been back to see her doctor, who offered little assistance. (Unfortunately, he was also a relative, so she hesitated to seek a second opinion.) As I suspected, she had been sewn up too tightly with the "husband's knot." Even gentle pressure to the area caused bleeding, as the skin tore ever so slightly apart. Both she and her partner were frustrated and miserable, and eventually, she had to have reconstructive surgery. But other women who have seen me for this problem report spontaneous resolution with application of evening primrose oil to the perineum, massaged in thoroughly twice a day.

Bleeding without pain is normal for up to six weeks, but it should be fairly light from three weeks on. It may increase temporarily with intense physical activity, indicating a need for more rest. The first lovemaking may also cause some bleeding, which is perfectly normal. But bleeding that persists past six weeks might indicate that placental fragments have been retained or the endometrium has overproliferated. If there is any doubt, it's best to see your care provider.

A major concern heterosexual women have about resuming sex is whether they will have sufficient vaginal tone to satisfy their partner. Some tone is usually lost with the birth, although breast-feeding naturally helps to restore it. Pelvic floor exercises can be resumed as early as the first day postpartum. These aren't particularly easy at first, but they may feel more natural and effective if done while breast-feeding (linking them to a particular activity also makes it easier to remember to do them).

There are three basic pelvic floor exercises that I recommend. The first tones the vault of the vagina; it is known as the "elevator exercise." Relax your muscles completely, then draw them up, one "floor" at a time. Hold the position for a few moments at the top, then let your muscles down again floor by floor, all the way to the "basement." The second exercise tones the side walls of the vagina and fine-tunes tone in the vault. Relax completely, then, pulling upward again, make a longitudinal stroking motion within the vagina, as if you were caressing a soft fruit and squeezing out the juice. The third exercise tones the bulbocavernosus muscle near the vaginal opening. Again, relax completely, then quickly contract low in the vagina with quick, snapping movements. Do as many repetitions as you can, then increase day by day. If you are unsure of what you are doing or whether you are making progress, put your fingers inside and find out. These movements are sacred to both Tantric and Kundalini traditions, whereby women initiate the flow of sexual energy up the spine and throughout the body to experience bliss and enlightenment. These movements also occur naturally with orgasm, so sex itself is a great way to retone the vagina.

Here are several accounts of first sex postpartum that serve to illustrate both the awkwardness and the transformation possible at this time. From Tessa:

> John and I had been through so much with the birth, which we planned for home but ended up having in the hospital. There were complications, for me and the baby,

but I managed to give birth without needing a Cesarean. Then we had to stay in the hospital because of concerns for our son, and my husband was totally drawn into taking care of everything. He was down in the nursery when they needed to do tests, talking to the staff, protecting the baby, and bringing him right back to me. When we got home we were utterly exhausted, but that very night we made love. I knew I shouldn't—it was only the third day—but we couldn't help it, we had to reunite, the urge was irresistible. It was, I think, the most intimate and explosive sex we've ever had—it just burst from both of us. We had been so close in pregnancy, and we really reached deep for each other to get back to ourselves and heal what happened with the birth. I had a little bleeding after, but it was worth it . . . I'll never forget it.

From Julia:

I love Maria more than ever after the birth, to be with her and cuddle with the baby is just the best! We waited a couple weeks until she felt okay—she didn't have stitches or anything, and it was lovely to be able to feel inside her again. I was a bit tentative at first, but I knew she would be honest with me as we went along.

And from Christine:

I waited a full four weeks, and Jarred was at his limit. I hadn't been to the doctor yet, but I'd been looking in a mirror and feeling around, and everything seemed fine. Well, when he got inside me it felt so different that I think it shocked us both. The part that had stitches felt numb and stiff, and the rest of me felt all loose and out of control. But Jarred kept saying I felt so good, so warm, so soft that I put my fears aside and let myself go. Then I came, milk started spurting from my breasts, and the baby woke up and started crying like it somehow got the signal. I brought it into bed to nurse while Jarred licked milk from my other nipple—not exactly what I'd expected, but pretty satisfying all in all.

Leaking milk, by the way, is normal with orgasm because of the letdown stimulating effects of oxytocin. As for the baby waking at the exact moment of orgasm, it's been noted that prolactin tends to synchronize mother-infant sleep cycles, causing a kind of physiological empathy between the two.

This brings us to yet another area of concern, that of sleeping arrangements for the baby. In the last few decades, family sleeping—baby or children in bed with their parents—has seen a surge of popularity in this country. Reports from those who have tried it are somewhat mixed but basically positive. At least in the beginning, having the baby in bed makes a big difference in how much sleep the mother gets; often, she is able to nurse without fully awakening. The risk of rolling on top of the baby has proven to be just a myth, and increased skin-to-skin intimacy has emotional benefits for both parents and child. However, if it gets to the point where you and your partner are sleeping in separate beds, it's time to reconsider the arrangement.

A wise pediatrician friend suggests that right from the start, parents put the baby on its own little mattress (or in a bassinet) next to their bed, at least for part of the night. This may help the baby get used to sleeping alone, if only part time. One mother relayed that after a particularly difficult night, she and her partner decided to move their ten-month-old daughter to another room, and she suddenly began sleeping through the night. Apparently she had been disturbed by her parents' noises. But the mother also noted that this was not a permanent arrangement; in a few weeks, her daughter was back sleeping with them again. Sleeping all night in solitude is uncommon for little ones; children may climb into their parents' bed in the wee hours of the morning for many years to come.

How does this work in terms of sex? It depends on the age of the child; if yours is still an infant and you find yourself interrupted in the middle of something sweet, you may wish to quietly continue. Many women report the stopgap solution of nursing the baby while making love: an odd juggle of emotions, but eminently practical.

Your toddler will probably be a bit too aware for this sort of thing. Still, be sure to let your little one see you and your partner cozily together, hugging and kissing, lest this behavior lead to anxiety should she or he come upon you unawares. Of course, any child will be less jealous and possessive if regularly given lots of love and affection.

Ultimately, new parents make do. And they become creative, seeking out different times and places for an intimate rendezvous. See the forthcoming section, "Recapturing Intimacy," for further suggestions.

Sexual Inhibition and Dysfunction

Sometimes, sexuality is affected by more than the usual emotional adjustments or practical concerns. Any serious setback in physical recuperation, or a traumatic event like the death of a loved one, the loss of a job, or a sudden need to relocate can have a major effect on libido.

If it has not already surfaced, deep-seated ambivalence about gender roles may arise in the father. If he is harboring the old Madonna/Whore dichotomy, this may be the breaking point. Perhaps he was able to love his partner well enough during the pregnancy, but now finds himself deeply uncomfortable relating to her as a mother. She may notice that he seems hesitant to touch her and think it's because her looks have changed, or she is no longer sexually enticing, while the real reason is his own internal conflict. Some men respond to this by having affairs; others plunge into their work or some recreational activity. Either way, life suffers at home, and intervention is called for. Bear in mind that the postpartum period may be the first—and undoubtedly the most critical—time for a man to face up to misogynist attitudes and beliefs at odds with his better judgment. There is nothing easy about this process, but it can lead in the long run to more intimate ways of living and loving.

For herself, a woman may feel confused and frustrated in the conflicting roles of mother, lover, and career woman. As long as she reassures her partner that these conflicts have nothing whatsoever to do with his or her adequacy, they will have a chance at intimacy. She may find, however, that she must set new boundaries—something of a taboo for women in this culture. Yet personal boundaries are essential for healthy relationships. A new mother desperately needs to conserve her energy, muster her strength repeatedly, and say no to anything that conflicts with her instincts. Setting boundaries means being straightforward, not holding back. Key phrases include "I can't. Could you . . . ?"; "No, not right now"; "Could we talk about it later?"; and finally, "I need to get some rest."

In the same vein, it is important to be realistic about sex in this phase; it's not going to be like it was before. The combination of bone-weary fatigue, interruptions from the baby, and worry about finances, household matters, and work schedules is hardly conducive to joyous and spontaneous lovemaking. This simply is not one of those honeymoon times in a couple's life when sex is a breeze. This needn't cause panic, though, if both partners can keep their perspective and remember that this phase is only temporary. This is really what intimate partnership is all about—keeping the long view and loving as much as we can along the way.

Sylvia reports:

> I felt very estranged from my body and so tired all the time I didn't want sex at all. But Mark would put pressure on me. Then I'd get in the mood, and he'd be too worn out, worried or something. Finally, I got in the habit of shutting him out, until one day he broke down and told me how much he missed me, missed our closeness. Really, I had forgotten that he cared, that I cared. The birth just turned me upside down, I guess, and I was so involved with the baby.
>
> I told him what it was like for me, how exhausted and used up I felt, and as we talked, one thing led to another and we were making love. It sure wasn't perfect (the baby actually interrupted with a nursing) but it was real. You know that quality, when sex is ultra-real? It was raw, it was different, it was new—we were three now, instead of two, more instead of less. Once I saw this, staying connected to Mark became easier. We got really good at blending sex into ordinary, day-to-day things we did, so that when we were alone, we got intimate right away. I felt like I had discovered the secret to a happy marriage and wondered, "How come no one ever told me about this?"

When we learn to support each other in spite of stress, or even because of it, our sexual experience takes on deeper meaning. When we make love in order to learn and grow, when we can set aside our expectations and take from sex whatever we find, we have entered a new stage of sexual maturity. The challenges of the postpartum period naturally initiate this evolution.

Recapturing Intimacy

Ideally, intimacy is not seriously interrupted or lost in the process of giving birth. But there is change, as discussed, and sometimes a couple must work to reestablish closeness and trust. This means talking about sex, communicating hurts, fears, and desires more openly than ever. With a baby around, it also means making an effort to be emotionally and sexually available to each other, even when one partner is not fully in the mood. It means picking up where you leave off, even though days may intervene, by keeping your intimacy alive in heart and deed.

Remember that you cannot have deep intimacy in relationship unless you find time to be intimate with yourself. Time alone is not a luxury; it is a necessity! You do not have to have a hot date with your partner or some important business errand to justify hiring a babysitter or asking a relative to watch the baby for a few hours. Use this time for yourself lovingly—relax, check in on your feelings, do something pleasurable or inspiring, be in touch with your soul's purpose.

Here are a few well-seasoned tips for keeping the fires burning:

1. Have some ritual in your sex life. Choose a night once a week to have dinner, wine, and watch a video after the baby is asleep, then have sex right there on the floor, on the couch, in the spare bedroom, or wherever takes your fancy. Even if you are interrupted and can't resume, you know your next special evening is only a week away.

2. Get out. Find a good babysitter willing to commit herself to a certain night each week. Choose someone you know and trust or seek recommendations from friends. It makes a difference to go out regularly: the benefits build up. Once out, you will tend to talk mostly about the baby, but try to talk about yourselves, too.

3. Make cooking and housework as easy as possible. If you ever planned to treat yourself to hired help, now is definitely the time to do it. Buy a slow cooker for meals that practically cook themselves, or resort to the microwave. I recommend that all pregnant women farm out dinner preparation for the first two weeks postpartum by enlisting every friend or relative who offers assistance or wants to come see the baby. Or, you can cook casseroles and soups in advance and freeze as much as possible.

4. Insist on time alone. This is time for your spirit, time you make sacred by having fun, renewing yourself, making sure you are well from the inside out. Start doing this now, and don't ever stop! And don't let anyone interrupt you or make you feel guilty, either, about taking this much-needed time for yourself.

5. Develop a sense of humor. If you don't have one already, you will definitely need it in the years ahead. Let your troubles roll off your shoulders. Joke around with your partner, your kids, yourself. Call good friends for a chat and some silliness. Let your heart be light, and look on the bright side of difficult situations.

6. Try not to burden your partner with grim realities, at least not on the emotional level. If you can translate your troubles into specific needs/instructions, okay, but otherwise, forget it. Take responsibility for what you feel. Try to find your own ways of alleviating stress and making yourself feel better. Find others to talk to for solace and inspiration.

7. Know that this wild and crazy time will pass. Maintain the long view, plan your first weekend (or weeklong) getaway with pleasure, and keep the faith.

Against all odds, many women feel their sexuality to be greatly enhanced by giving birth. Some have orgasms for the first time in their lives. Perhaps this is because birth partners a woman primarily with herself—the keys to letting go and making progress in labor come from within her. Especially if she has been buffeted around by male needs, desires, and opinions about sex, birth can be quite a revelation. As Cassie says:

> I never had orgasms like I did after giving birth. When I was pushing my daughter out, I was more than connected to my vaginal muscles—I actually became them. My strength was incredible, my timing exquisite. Before, when I made love it was me up here, vagina down there. But now my awareness and intelligence are fully inside me. I'm not afraid to do or try anything with my body; its power belongs to me. Once you've let go giving birth, letting go with sex can take you to places you've never dreamed of.

New Mother

◎

A week after our child was born,
you cornered me in the spare room
and we sank down on the bed.
You kissed me and kissed me, my milk undid its
burning slip-knot through my nipples,
soaking my shirt. All week I had smelled of milk,
fresh milk, sour. I began to throb:
my sex had been torn easily as cloth by the
crown of her head, I'd been cut with a knife and
sewn, the stitches pulling at my skin—
and the first time you're broken, you don't know
you'll be healed again, better than before.
I lay in fear and blood and milk
while you kissed and kissed me, your lips hot and swollen
as a teen-age boy's, your sex dry and big,
all of you so tender, you hung over me,
over the nest of the stitches, over the
splitting and tearing, with the patience of someone who
finds a wounded animal in the woods
and stays with it, not leaving its side
until it is whole, until it can run again.

From *The Dead and the Living* by Sharon Olds (New
York: Alfred Knopf, 1984).

chapter
six

Sex and Superwomen: The Myth of "Having It All"

Women of today are beyond busy. We precariously juggle the demands of our work, our primary relationships, our children, our friendships, and our own personal needs. Particularly if partnered with men, we continue to do the majority of the housework: running errands, paying bills, purchasing food and clothing, supervising household repairs, doing the cooking and laundry. We confer with our children's teachers and help with homework on a regular basis. If we are lucky, once in a while we lunch with a friend. If we happen to be self-employed, or are struggling to advance in our career, we are definitely in deep water!

Most women no longer have a choice about working outside the home. Even if we are partnered, our economy has thoroughly adapted to the two-income family. This has been true for some time now, long enough to give us a chance to assess the quality of our hectic lifestyles. We find that our needs for rejuvenation are increasingly swept aside for greater productivity. Few of us practice genuine rituals of self-care. We are lucky to be at work on time, survive the day's annoyances, handle personal business, and get dinner on the table. Later, we collapse into bed with little energy to talk or touch. Most of us barely get by each day, let alone find time for pleasure and intimacy.

Is there no way out of this dilemma? Before we can realistically discuss the effect of the superwoman syndrome on sexuality, we must realize how incompatible the two really are. In so many ways, lack of time to care for ourselves negates our sexual desire.

Of course, there are stopgap measures like the weekend getaway, lunch-break rendezvous, or quiet evening in. These do help to maintain a sense of balance by providing relief from tension. But ultimately, snatched moments together are not enough, because real intimacy cannot be staged or forced; it must be based on genuine and deep communication. If communication is continually fragmented, disrupted, or shelved indefinitely, sudden episodes of private time can end up in arguments or long, involved discussions that sap rather than renew us. As Margaret reported:

> We'd start out with a romantic meal or something, then wild and crazy sex. But when we finally got down to talking later, all that emerged was frustration and resentment. I just don't get it—why do I have to do it all? The daily routine is bad enough, but even when I'm supposedly free, I'm initiating talks and fielding the upsets. I feel unseen, invisible. I'm taking care of everything and everybody, but nobody cares for me.

Transforming Gender-Based Expectations

Margaret's lament hits it right on the mark for many of us. Unfortunately, the solution isn't any easier to bear than the problem, but here it is: the only one who can really take care of Margaret is Margaret herself. She must revamp her priorities so that her own are at the top. Further, her entire gender role must be recast from serving others to nurturing herself. This is a drastic shift from what our mothers believed and what society continues to expect of us.

This is especially difficult in that society refuses to accord women equal rights and privileges to those held by men. Men as a group have a higher pay scale, greater social security benefits, more free time, and more opportunity to play than women. With our role of servant so deeply entrenched in social structure, in the institutions of marriage, education, health care, business, and religion, we are going to have to assert loud and clear just exactly what we need, and how and when we need it. To again quote the indomitable Camille Paglia, "Feminism begins at home. It begins with every single woman drawing the line."[1] At first, this seems like just another job to do. But this is a worthwhile task, one that can cause inappropriate or demeaning roles to fall by the wayside; this is the key to our revolution. If men, women, and children are not equal in their basic human rights, our world will continue to be plagued with war, famine, disease, and poverty. The need to assert ourselves is more than a personal issue; it is a political, social, and ecological imperative.

Here is a quote from Sedonia Cahill, author of *Wisdom Circles*:

> It is nearly impossible not to get stuck in mothering in our society. That's certainly the role that the culture prefers, as far as I can tell. Women's basic and very good impulse to mother children has been so exploited by the patriarchy that they end up being mother to grown men, who are free to behave like children and become very boring. It's a major cause of dissension between men and women, this exploitation—there's such a pull to keep us locked into that place.
>
> To break out of being defined as a nurturer, a woman has to commit to her own life, and doing that is scary—choosing yourself instead of someone else is really a frightening thing to do, like you're being a bad girl. But even as a mother, you have to make a commitment to your own life. And I don't think that can be done without a circle of sisters, where you learn to feel good and wonderful about yourself, see yourself reflected in the eyes of women that you love very much—it helps you decide you are worth it, that your own life really must come first."[2]

For years, women were taught to be peacemakers, to soothe and field the emotional problems of others, to the exclusion of their own. When we behave this way with men, it's no wonder that we find them to be out of touch with their feelings. It is true that men have biolog-ical difficulties, due to brain structure and function, in linking emotion to other aspects of behavior and response. But why should we go so far as to translate their emotions for them? Perhaps we would find less resentment on their part if we focused our efforts on putting our feelings, needs, and desires forward overtly, rather than covertly. This is a different model of relationship than what most of us have imprinted, but it could serve to create a healthier sort of intimacy.

One woman shared these words from her husband: "You know, you women think you have it so hard, but at least you know what you're fighting for. You've got principles—for us guys, if we start to open up and change, it's pretty confusing." Although we may feel compassion for men in this quandary, we must continuously beware of our tendency to rescue them. When we do, we perpetuate the problem by colluding with it.

Women have been accused of late of being angry and reactive, but so are men. Our anger is easy to root in inequality, overwork, and unsupportive social structures; in short, we are angry at society. For men, society is basically supportive and therefore not the target, but women frequently are. Rape is obvious evidence of this; violent pornography further serves to illustrate. Men are angry with women for brushing them off, abandoning them to their own confusion, failing to make the pain and frustration of life easier to bear. And it's true that many of us are just too busy to bother with male angst as we once did.

On the other hand, the stress of competing in a man's world has led certain women to adopt male characteristics almost to the exclusion of their own. So deeply have we rebelled against being stereotyped as weak, indecisive, and irrational that some of us have inadvertently rejected the positive side of these aspects: the sensitivity, flexibility, and creativity to discern and chart our own course. True, we have virtually been forced to do so to advance in our careers. But perhaps the time has come to reincorporate these feminine aspects of our personalities into our way of life, our approach to problem solving, our intimate relationships.

In his book *Men, Women and Relationships*, John Gray describes four typical patterns of heterosexual partnership. Of particular relevance here is the pattern in which a woman becomes so independent that she severs critical ties with herself and others. We know her by the following: (1) she is overly defensive; (2) she is compulsively organized and responsible; (3) she is suspicious, cold, and critical; (4) she is pushy and manipulative; (5) she is tense, intolerant, judgmental, and impatient; and (6) she is unable to accept support.[3] Not surprisingly, she tends to be partnered to a man who is weak, dependent, and unfocused. It is easy to see how many of the brightest and most creative women of our time have ended up this way. But this unnatural, constricted state of being is clearly at odds with a woman's chances for health and happiness, sexual pleasure, and intimacy.

As Stacy relates, "I kept blaming Bob, but I knew it was me. I had become so sharp with him, so on edge all the time, so critical and controlling, that we just didn't get along. I convinced myself that sex was still fine; after all, I knew exactly how to let my guard down in bed. But the chemistry between us, the erotic side of our day-to-day contact, was missing."

Similarly, men who have sought to subdue their masculine traits in deference to the feminine may find themselves less dynamic in their relationships or life in general. Although it's good for men to be open, sensitive, and easygoing at times, chronic confusion, indecisiveness, or irresponsibility are signs of trouble. Particularly when a man begins to live on dreams, or becomes moody and withdrawn much of the time, something is definitely wrong.

With male and female aspects out of balance, sex will invariably be affected, because the fundamental attraction between opposites has been disrupted. Perhaps the most common mistake in relationships is trying to make our partners more like ourselves, more manageable and predictable. As our differences diminish, so will the attraction. We turn into good friends instead of lovers; the passion is gone. Gray states, "To whatever extent a partner must suppress their ways of being, feeling, thinking, or doing in order to receive love or be safe in a relationship, the passion will fade."

This is a complex matter and not easy to remedy. In general, women can benefit by recognizing and owning both their feminine and masculine traits and keeping an eye on the balance. Women today often need to deliberately evoke the feminine by circling with other women and airing pressing issues in their lives. Changes in lifestyle, in the daily blend of activity and rest, may also be called for, and sometimes the only way to accomplish this is by breaking routine or taking a vacation. Fine-tuning the male and female in oneself can be a lot of fun, and to be able to do so is a landmark of maturity, bound to have an enriching effect on sexuality.

In any event, we women need intimate relationships in our lives. We are generally so expansive by nature, so relational that we lose ourselves in others without giving it a thought. Yet our intimate links with others can also help us reconnect with ourselves. Remember that women generally prefer to solve problems by talking matters through with their friends, formulating and evolving their thoughts aloud. This unique ability of women to share half-baked truths, in contrast to men's preference for airing already polished positions, has been referred to by women themselves as "real talk."[4] It is time we acknowledge that certain of our needs readily met by women are rarely satisfied by men.

Let us return to the importance of circling for women. As women advance in their thirties, they begin to recognize the power of menstruation in their lives and to truly appreciate their cyclic round of moods and aptitudes each month. Most settle into a regular rhythm, and many notice that synchronous cycling with their co-workers or housemates has become fairly consistent. As they approach their forties, they may begin to celebrate their joint moon time, comparing notes and deliberately going deeper into their revelations. When discussing indigenous societies, we refer to this as entrainment. Menstrual entrainment is the basis for what I term "blood bonding" — that is, the deep interconnectedness of women who intentionally share their menstrual wisdom and vision to unite with one another. Blood bonding takes women's circling up a notch; it makes possible a level of work and play heretofore unknown to most women.

What does this have to do with revamping gender-based expectations? The stronger women are in their own ways of knowing and being, the less inclined they are to fuss and worry about their differences with men. If asked, most men say that they wish women would speak to them calmly, giving them clear and simple instructions rather than process or diatribe. This gives us an important hint on why women need to circle, and how circling can, albeit indirectly, improve our relationships with men.

Nevertheless, major shifts in gender-based expectations carry the liability of loss, whether loss of identity in the relationship, of familiar patterns of interaction, or of sexual intimacy. These losses are usually temporary, but they can be worrisome.

Susan reveals:

> When I started to be truthful with my partner about what I needed, I was pretty scared. Scared he wouldn't love me, wouldn't care, or even worse, couldn't help me. We were both surprised, I think, to find that our relationship actually endured, and things began to change for the better. But for a while, we couldn't make love. A lot was being stirred up for both of us.

If estrangement persists in a relationship, the underlying issues must be identified. A couple might be able to manage this on their own, or they may need the help of a professional. In any event, when dealing with shifts in gender roles, a little patience goes a long way—it can give both parties a chance to stretch, experiment, grow, and reach new depths of understanding essential for any long-term solution.

Sex and Anger

On the other hand, if there is deep-seated anger in relationship, sexual intimacy will all but vanish. As expert Marilyn Ruman, Ph.D., says, "Anger is almost always the enemy of desire and is one of the best places to look when your sex life is floundering."[5]

Unfortunately, anger is often repressed or unconscious in relationships. Typically, one partner will try to force the other to act the anger out, while taking a turn at resistance and avoidance. These patterns usually have roots in a childhood spent with parents doing much the same, enacting extremes of submission and domination. Particularly when chemical dependency, physical abuse, or sexual abuse are part of the family story, a survivor comes to believe (and rightly so, in such situations) that expressing anger leads to danger and unhappiness.

An unhealthy relationship to anger is also endemic of patriarchy, with its hierarchical structure of privilege based on "power over" rather than "power with" others. In truth, anger is a natural emotion, nothing to feel ashamed of. It's what we do with it that counts. If we enact patriarchal values by using our anger to try to control others, we miss its real purpose in our lives—to spur us to take a stand against injustice, cruelty, and violence.

The shadow side of anger is sadness and loss. If there are unresolved traumas in the family history that have filtered into the relationship, they must be worked through before there can be any hope for intimacy. Time is of the essence, though, especially for the relationship in which anger has been repressed but is now beginning to explode. The longer a couple has been holding back and accumulating resentment, the more each will expect—or will try to force—the other to make it up to them. This can lead to various forms of abuse and also serves to illustrate why patterns of dependency and abuse tend to be self-perpetuating.

One way to work with occasional anger is to recognize that it correlates to need. It is important to acknowledge our anger, yes, but it is even more critical (and functional) to articulate the need it represents. If a couple can agree to deal with anger as it arises by making time to hear each other's needs and attempting either to meet them or to negotiate alternatives, intimacy may soon resurface.

It may also be necessary to weed out patterns of avoidance in the relationship. Spending inordinate amounts of time in separate parts of the house, taking meals separately, going to bed at different times, or arguing just before bed are classic examples of repressed anger, as are not taking care of oneself physically, neglecting shared environments (particularly the bedroom), or cluttering free time with small talk and busywork. Deliberate changes in these areas can prompt discussion, but should this escalate to confrontation that only makes matters worse, professional help is called for.

Stress and Sexuality

Stress, too, is an enemy of desire. Consider the physical effects of stress on the body, particularly on the adrenal glands. The adrenals have two parts, the medulla and the cortex. When we are stressed, the medulla produces catecholamines, one of which is adrenaline, responsible for our flight-or-fight response when threatened or under fire. The cortex is responsible for producing the sex hormones estrogen and progesterone, but more significantly, the testosterone responsible for the libido. To some degree these functions are opposing; for example, if stress is chronic or protracted so that the medulla must continually pump the body with catecholamines, androgen production from the cortex may be neglected. Here we have a physiological explanation of how stress may dampen sexual desire.

Psychologically, stress causes us either to fight or to withdraw. Sexual activity under these circumstances simply may not occur, or it may be brief and fairly explosive. Nothing wrong with the latter, except that it precludes the comfort and intimacy essential in any long-term relationship. The situation is even more difficult if both partners are under stress. The challenges of trying to unwind in bed, encountering emotions carefully held in check while trying to coordinate with another doing the same, can be uncomfortable enough to dissuade both from making another effort.

Some couples manage nonsexual phases by keeping the communication going in other ways, particularly through shared activities that both enjoy. Others choose to have sex—whether good, bad, or indifferent—to maintain some degree of connection. Either way, couples suffering from chronic stress will find it an obstacle to intimacy. The answer lies not in the bedroom, but in coming to terms with the problem and responding to it intelligently. From Natalie:

> It's rough for us right now: we both knock ourselves out at work, the kids get little of our attention, we both feel guilty and angry, and we often take it out on each other. Then we have sex to make up. Sometimes it's great, a real release. Sometimes it just doesn't make it; we're still all bottled up, and we feel more separate than before. But that's marriage, I guess.

To complicate matters, men and women generally have different reactions to stress. Whereas men tend to withdraw to consider the situation, women respond with a rush of emotion, wanting more than anything else to sift through their feelings and discuss them in order to find some stability. This is the only way most women can separate their needs from the needs of others and avoid becoming overwhelmed.

Women who are overwhelmed have one characteristic in common: they lose the ability to prioritize.[6] Every task and obligation suddenly assumes equal importance. Whether it's finishing up a project on a deadline or loading the dishwasher, everything is done in a continuous overwrought stream of activity, rather like a runaway train.

The more a woman becomes overwhelmed, the more likely she is to overreact to the inconsequential. Not being able to distinguish the important issues, she will find little irritations and focus her frustration and anger on them. Every woman knows the idiotic feeling of exploding in fury over the unwashed dishes in the sink or the single paper napkin scuttling about the floor. At this point, total exhaustion is forthcoming. She feels utterly drained, useless, and alone. This scenario takes its toll on everyone who loves her.

When we hit bottom, we see clearly that the long-suffering, self-negating approach to stress and its causes does not work. Unfortunately, we often forget this lesson as we reemerge from the depths—we try to normalize quickly, put on a happy face, and get back to work, only to have the pattern repeat itself once more. This is because our culture teaches us to fear the depths, to equate the experience of falling apart and hitting bottom with psychosis and/or depression. When we go deep into the well of being, we cease to be available to others and are no longer "productive." Yet this process, known as "descent" in numerous spiritual traditions, is really a sacred one.

Descent gives us the opportunity to rest, not in the void, as we might fear, but in the holy womb of the Great Mother, the matrix of creation. If we fully surrender, we may experience great insight and rejuvenation that stays with us as we ascend. But if we fight our descent or try to reemerge before we are ready, we miss the point and are apt to be plagued with anxiety or bouts of true depression.

Here is a quote from Adele Getty, author of *A Sense of the Sacred*:

> The image I had of myself was of being on a large, black sea, madly flailing around like a many-armed goddess, every arm flailing on the surface of the water as I tried to stay afloat. Finally, in the midst of this panic I called for help and said, "What is this about and what can I do? This is taking a lot of energy, trying to stay afloat." I couldn't sleep, and no matter what I tried to do during the day, psychically I was flailing. And this voice just came and said, "Surrender, just drown, just let go and drown." I stopped flailing and I let myself drown—and I drowned, but I didn't die. I sank into his sea of peace, calmness, serenity . . . no, serenity is too strong . . . it didn't have the positive energy serenity has, but there was nothing negative about it. It was emptiness, and it wasn't taking any energy anymore and it was alright, I could just be there in this emptiness. It wasn't blissful but I could sleep, and immediately the energetics of my life shifted and started supporting me again. But if I tried to jump in with both feet, pick up the ball and run with it, I immediately got smashed back down. A month would go by and I'd think, "Surely I can start being actively engaged in this process," but nope, I'd be wrong . . . and this went on for nine months. My natural tendency is to bob back up and start running, but the challenge was not to emerge too soon from the underworld. Making the descent is a process, being in the underworld is a process, and making the ascent, slowly coming back is a process too, and if you short circuit any step along the way, you're going to have to go though the journey again.[7]

On the other hand, if stress and the trauma it causes are chronic due to illness, unemployment, addiction, or other long-term crisis involving a loved one or family member, outside help is essential. There may be no immediate solution, but at least the difficulty can be tempered with support.

When in high-stress situations like these, we must continue to care for and nurture ourselves, as this is the only way we can possibly meet the challenges of caring for others. Beyond support, we need our own outside activities, some structure and routine, meaningful work to do. Sex may be low on the list of priorities; certainly this makes sense from a physiological standpoint. Or, with intention, it may serve as the glue that keeps us together if we find ourselves in dire straits.

How Children Affect Sexuality

For those who have children, let's look at how family life can influence sexuality. We will begin with an overview of the key developmental phases in children's lives, and how these might affect a woman's inclination for and enjoyment of sex.

T. Berry Brazelton, authority on child rearing and development, says that when a child reaches the age of two, the parents may begin to compete for his or her affections.[8] If competition or poor communication exist in other areas of their lives—which is quite likely, considering how little time parents of a toddler have for themselves and each other—they may become sexually estranged. For want of privacy and intimacy, parents may inadvertently transfer their needs onto their child and vie bitterly for his or her attention.

If this situation is left unaddressed, studies show that the likelihood of extramarital affairs is high, reaching a peak when the child is three or four. Once the couple is past this critical point, the survival issues of the first few years have been surmounted—and parents have an opportunity to view the wreckage. If there is ever a time when parents need and deserve a vacation for themselves, it is now.

Here are some practical suggestions that might help to forestall such a crisis.

Take Private Time

Again, this is not optional! It is the only way to find the energy to relate intimately to your partner. Try to squeeze a bit of time out of your usual routine. Simplify meals so you have free time before dinner. Do household chores in chunks, running several tasks simultaneously to save time and steps. Lower your standards for neatness and cleanliness, to save not only time but your nerves.

A more lasting approach is to change your routines so that time for yourself is built in. Right from the start, teach your children ways to take care of themselves. Those of us whose parents tried to give us the best of everything may need to unlearn certain self-sacrificing behaviors. We must create a healthier model of family life, wherein every member does his or her share. In heterosexual unions, this typically means teaching your partner how to care for himself, as well as to perform his share of household duties. If you are in a position to hire additional help, do it. Save your relationship by taking care of yourself first and foremost.

Sociologist Pepper Schwartz of the University of Washington identifies three types of marriage arrangements: (1) traditional marriage; (2) near-peer marriage; and (3) peer marriage. Traditional marriage is that wherein husband and wife play conventional roles, with sharply divided tasks and responsibilities. In a near-peer marriage, both spouses have jobs, but the wife still does the majority of the housework and child rearing. Peer marriages are fully egalitarian matches; each spouse has equal rank and is responsible for both the economic and emotional well-being of the household, with chores divided equally. Partners in peer marriages report an intense sense of companionship and high levels of intimacy.[9]

Housework is such a charged issue for most couples that it deserves a few more words. As regards keys to an enduring marriage, author Andrew Ward dryly advises, "It doesn't matter if one of you spends all day on the patio eating bonbons, you've got to divide housework right down the middle. Actual equalized work schedules, impervious to the shirker and martyr among you (shirkers and martyrs compose most married couples), should be hammered out right away and signed, preferably in blood, by both parties."[10]

Keep Up with Your Dreams

Don't let your dreams fade so that you no longer remember them. Take time to review your goals in life and your fantasies of what could be, giving yourself the freedom to be visionary. Where do you want to be a year from now, or five, or ten years hence? What must you absolutely do in life to feel you have really lived? Some say that whatever you loved to do most when age seven or eight holds a key to your future. Think back, dream forward, and keep track of what you see.

Make Time for the Relationship

When you are very busy, intimacy must be made a priority. This means setting aside "couple time," literally scheduling it in. Maintain a regular weekly date night. And set aside another time, preferably in the morning when you are both fresh, to talk about what is going on in your lives and how you are feeling. This time of open disclosure works best if you both agree to hear each other out without being judgmental. Some couples do this daily, others once a week, but the more you practice, the more it will occur spontaneously.

Never underestimate the power of an entire night alone together. There is a dramatic difference between sex when you know you might be interrupted and sex with total privacy. Plus, it's nice to have the freedom to resume again later in the evening if you feel like it. At least twice a year, make plans to get away to some romantic location. When you are busy with family life, you must work to re-create your love.

Surprise Yourself and Your Lover

Do the unexpected once in a while. When your love was young, it was exciting to try new things together, share adventures, discover your commonalities in a variety of situations. Let this element of excitement back into your life, and don't worry about appearing foolish. Take a few risks on new activities, and update your style to reflect your growth. Often, we marry (or make long-term commitments) because we want stability; we long for a nice, simple routine. But routine is routine—it needs the spice of innovation to keep it from becoming dull. Reanimate yourself with new experiences, new impressions. This is a time-honored way of stimulating creativity and passion.

Get Help If You Need It

Marriage or couple counseling doesn't have to be a long-term proposition. People often end up in counseling because it is the only way they seem able to make the time to talk to one another. The main benefit of counseling is that it provides an opportunity to be witnessed. Someone who is objective about your problems can reframe them in ways that make it easier for you to handle them on your own. Almost every intimate partnership needs a boost like this once in a while.

A critical period for mothers is that when their child begins school full-time. The child is no longer fully dependent, and all the trappings of that phase come to an end. The mother who has been free to stay at home will suddenly have lots of time during the day—so much that she may be at a loss for ways to fill it. On the other hand, the mother who has been unable to spend much time with her child may feel longing for the irreplaceable phase she has missed. These emotions may be difficult to explain to one's partner, because they are closely linked to the mother-infant bond—though increasingly, men (or women) who provide close care in the early years have these feelings too. But those not so intimately involved tend to dismiss these empty-nest blues as the height of irrationality. They remember the sleepless nights, the mad shuffle for babysitters, the interrupted lovemaking, and above all, their partner's complaints, and then wonder how she can possibly be serious.

Nevertheless, this juncture is one when mothers must reassemble their identity and establish new goals for themselves and their primary relationship. If you have been a full-time mom and suddenly have time on your hands, the questions are tough. What are you to do now? Who are you, with your child out of your arms and in school? Now is the time to recall your pre-motherhood ambitions. Particularly if you have given up your career for motherhood and are thinking of going back to work, you must take a hard look at how far you have fallen behind.

In any period of change, we use what we have been as a springboard for what we wish to become. Listen to what Christine has to say:

> I was happy Zoe was off to school, but I did feel a little empty. Especially with my husband—I just couldn't make him understand. Really, I didn't understand it myself, until one day it was suddenly clear. Before, when I was recovering from the birth and trying to get my body back, I wanted him to love me for what I was before—to remind me, you know? Now, with Zoe out in the world, I want him to reaffirm me for the mother I have become, and let me know I don't have to be anything else.

Again, we have an example of a woman wanting reassurance from her partner that she really needs to give to herself. It is important that we search our feelings for the seeds of our own direction and respond accordingly.

From ages five to seven, children identify with the family unit; thereafter they begin to relate to society at large. And then comes adolescence. Many mothers find their adolescent daughters to be particularly challenging. I recall describing mine at age eleven as being in "a perpetual state of PMS." This is the time when girls become extremely critical of their mothers, particularly as regards personal appearance. I remember coming down the stairs dressed for a party one night when my daughter remarked most caustically, "You're not going to wear *that*, are you?" The stress is compounded if Mom has reached a major chronological landmark of her own—say, her fortieth birthday. In spite of herself, she may end up making expensive trips to the cosmetics counter, beauty salon, or dieters group. Not that this is necessarily bad, but the upshot may be persisting uncertainty about her physical attractiveness.

The natural shift in power that occurs in adolescence may further complicate matters. Particularly if your parenting style has been to enforce your will on your young ones, their natural rebellion at this age can leave you feeling utterly powerless. And in truth, the role of parent does begin to change from director to guide and confidant. If you too are in upheaval, for whatever reason, this change in your role may feel like yet another blow to your self-confidence. This may merit counseling or professional help of some kind, as this is not a good time to be reactive or forceful with your children.

The "bread baking" approach to child rearing goes like this: You mix and add ingredients when children are young, you watch the dough rise (and must deflate it occasionally) as they mature, but once the bread is in the oven of adolescence, you had best not open the door! Sure, you keep an eye on things, but you don't interfere unless the bread is about to burn.

The Midlife Turnaround

◎

Superwomen and supermoms come in all ages. But depending on the decade of a woman's life, she will have particular sexual needs and orientation. Sex in young adulthood is largely about identifying with and pleasing another. Sex in the thirties tends to focus on pair-bonding and procreation. Sex in midlife reestablishes the priorities of the self: physical, emotional, and spiritual. Taking the long view, it makes sense that the tremendous push for security and success during our twenties and thirties might lead to a values and identity crisis in our forties. It should come as no surprise that a similar crisis might follow sexually.

Our cultural image of midlife crisis is that of older man, younger woman. This, from Barbara, illustrates how a woman in midlife can find meaning in weathering such an experience:

> My husband had affairs from the time he turned forty, and I only found out three years later. I was so furious, so humiliated that I really didn't think we were going to make it. Couldn't sleep with him at all, but he wanted to stay so we had counseling. All that stuff, I'll spare you—but when we finally started making love again, I was a different woman. I went out for myself. Whenever the pain of his betrayal would start to get to me, I'd hold on to myself and just do what I felt was best for me. I got in touch with a strength I didn't know I had before, and I aligned myself with it, even in bed.

Of course, there are many women who choose, with all good reason, to cut their losses on pain like this and move on. Some have affairs of their own, in search of healing. Others become obsessed with their attractiveness, doing almost anything to stay young. But what

Barbara referred to as aligning with her strength is increasingly crucial, as it enables us to meet challenges to our health and identity as we continue to age. Is it not therefore fitting that in midlife, we should seek to explore and express ourselves as never before? "Forty and fabulous": we know what we like, we speak our minds, we have a solid base from which to innovate, and pleasure is ours for the taking!

Here's an interesting comment from a friend a few weeks after her fortieth birthday:

> I thought midlife crises were only for men. But it's really hit me . . . I'm turning into a real loudmouth, saying things to my boss and husband I wouldn't have dreamed of saying before! You figure you have only so much time . . . I feel almost ruthless about getting my needs met.

And what was this doing to her sex life?

> This is pretty personal, but in the middle of making love one night I just blurted out, "Joe, why don't you *concentrate?*" I never said anything like that before . . . see, my husband just tends to ramble on sometimes in bed, without focusing on me. When he paused (I guess he was a little shocked), I added, "You know, concentrate on me." I couldn't believe I did that!

It is a well-known fact that whereas men reach their sexual peak (as per intensity and endurance) in their early twenties, women reach theirs later, often in their forties. This is partly physical, partly psychological. For many women, it takes that long to get to know themselves sexually, to overcome taboos of sexual self-expression, to come to know and trust their bodies, and to be confident enough to let go and get what they want in bed.

This is also a time when women who have never fantasized before find their sexual imagination coming to life. In her book *Women on Top*, author Nancy Friday makes clear both the range and the outrageousness of women's sexual fantasies as they reach this peak. Interestingly, these fantasies are quite physically oriented, focused on ways of maximizing sensation, while the fantasies of younger women are more emotionally based. For example, a woman in her twenties might fantasize about a long romantic buildup and tender preludes to lovemaking, whereas the midlife woman will focus more on sexual positions and her partner's techniques, or even on bondage and multiple partners as enhancements to her sensation.

June Reinisch, in "The Kinsey Report," notes that men and women do a turnaround in sexual temperament about this time. As women become more intrigued with physical experimentation, men become interested in letting themselves be vulnerable and caring.[11] These changes are hormonally based, for as women approach menopause, their reproductive hormones surge intensely to force ovulation. Thus, women tracking their cycles commonly report fertile peaks like never before, with ovulation so intense that, as one woman put it, "I'm wet down to my knees!" Testosterone levels also rise dramatically in women during their forties. But for men of the same age, testosterone begins gradually to decrease. In effect, women become more masculine, and men, more feminine. This explains a little-appreciated fact about men in midlife crisis: they tend to seek out younger women not so much for the wild reenactment of youthful passion, but because these women are sexually oriented precisely as they themselves wish to be, emotionally and romantically. This strikes women in their forties as the height of irony: all those years they yearned for romance, while he wanted nothing but sex! The trick is to turn these facts of life to one's advantage—which some women do by forming liaisons with younger men.

Testosterone levels do, in fact, correlate to degree of aggressiveness in women and, in many instances, to the inclination to stay in monogamous relationships. According to a study conducted by Patricia Schreiner-Engel, associate professor of obstetrics/gynecology and psychiatry at Mount Sinai School of Medicine in New York, women in the most powerful career positions had the highest testosterone levels and were extremely achievement-oriented. One was the head of a nursing union; another was an importer. Almost none of them were in an ongoing long-term relationship. On the other hand, women with lower testosterone levels were often homemakers, students, or temporary workers, and they tended to have enduring marriages.

Socioeconomic factors obviously affect these findings. But something very important, and heretofore overlooked, can be extrapolated from this research as regards women in midlife. If it is true that women at this stage experience the effects of skyrocketing testosterone linked to urges for independence, there must be a correlation between peak levels of this hormone and midlife crisis, not to mention the high divorce rate among couples in their forties.

All the more reason, then, for recasting sex roles and experimenting a little. In time, polarization will occur if there is no give and take in the relationship, or if the newly revised sexual needs of both partners are not being met.

Says Laurie:

> At first, I thought there was something wrong with my partner, that he was slowing down, losing his grip for some physical reason. This happened about the same time I seemed to want sex to be more physically forceful than before: faster, rougher, more intense. I found myself getting impatient with Ken, wishing he'd get on with it, at the same time feeling like a heel for being so pushy and demanding. But damn, what I wanted felt right to me, and I didn't want to put on the brakes.

This is a good start; the feeling is genuine and fits with the natural shift. But there will be a breakdown without frank communication, understanding, and mutual support. If he wants to take more time warming up, choose your favorite foreplay and spell it out, loud and clear. If he is pacing himself to the utmost, initiate changes in position that keep the stimulation level high enough for you. Bring your fantasies into the picture somehow. And don't be surprised if he is the one wanting afterglow cuddling and pillow talk!

The positive side of these changes is illustrated by these words from Candace:

> We'd been together for twelve years, and I finally felt like our sex life was fully on track. We truly understood where the other was coming from, because we'd each pretty much been there ourselves—we'd run the gamut I guess. Sex just got better and better, and we had an erotic dimension in our communication that I remembered from the early stages of our relationship. It surprised me, exceeded my expectations, and was well worth waiting for.

This may also be a time when women seek intimate relationships with other women for the first time, based on common needs and desires. As Lynn reports:

> I never considered myself bisexual, never thought of being with a woman until I reached a place of certainty and confidence in myself that made me long for the affinity of an equal. I'd been with so many men, struggling with their problems. Then I fell in love with Susan, and found common life experience, humor, flexibility, and passion perfect for this time of my life.

In the next chapter, we will look at the transformative effects of menopause on a woman's life and sexuality.

Sexual Transformation in Menopause

Opinions of menopause in our society are mixed at best. Not only does menopause signal the end of fertility, but it is notorious for its physical and emotional side effects. Hot flashes hit unexpectedly, vaginal dryness can be distressing, and mood swings make us scream and cry as if we were in our teens. If our difficulties in accepting "the change" lead us to fight against it, these side effects often become increasingly extreme.

Compounding menopausal symptoms is our cultural bias against aging—particularly toward women, who often find themselves bereft of identity as they grow older. No wonder we approach menopause with a sense of dread! But there are ways to view this passage that accord us greater dignity and self-respect so that its benefits, not the least of which are sexual, may be celebrated and enjoyed.

At age forty-eight, I was the first of my circle of women to enter menopause. This was difficult, because even though my sisters were close behind, I was constantly moving into uncharted territory and often felt isolated. Our discussions of menopause usually focused on our symptoms, with mutual suggestions for herbs, dietary changes, or comfort measures. Occasionally we'd talk about shifts in our sexuality, but with little clarity. We knew we were changing, but we didn't know how, and we certainly didn't know where we were going. After many months, I was finally able to verbalize my frustration: "I don't want to know about this remedy or that, I want to know what is happening to me!"

Before long, I became so alarmed by my explosive moods and shifting priorities that I decided to call for a Menopause Council in my community. There were five women I met with socially but didn't know well; they called themselves alternately "The Hot Potatoes," "The Fried Potatoes," or, "The Wild Yams." I asked one who was adept at women's circling if she would be willing to organize the council, and she agreed.

Soon I received an announcement for an event titled "The Other Side of Menopause." Each of the five organizers included a brief bio, and I was repeatedly struck by their third-person descriptions of how menopause had changed their lives:

> She stopped bleeding at fifty-two, flipped the dial, and started listening to Her Own Voice.

> She last bled when she was fifty-three and has been expressing Grandmother's Voice of Wisdom and Truth.

> She stopped bleeding at forty-two after her uterus was removed and has since plunged into the well of grief, amazed to find laughter there as well as tears.

> She stopped bleeding when she was fifty, walked through a menopause door and met herself, and has become "Queen of her Own Country."

> She last bled when she was fifty-one, is her own Wild Darling, and the Heroine of Her Own Story.

The effect of that council was far-reaching for me and for the forty other women who participated. Many of my fears were laid to rest, as I began to understand the scope of menopause as a major life change. I learned that my experience of feeling out of sync with normal responsibilities was common, and I was reassured that the physical and emotional turmoil I felt was healthy. I also began to see that the sexual revolution going on inside me actually had a purpose.

What Is Menopause?

Beyond the obvious symptom of cessation of the menses are the physical causes of menopause. At puberty, a girl has approximately three hundred thousand egg-forming cells, but a woman approaching menopause has only eight thousand or so follicles remaining. Over the years, her eggs have been destroyed by a combination of stress, radiation (exposure to the sun), and natural degeneration. As the eggs diminish in number, ovulation may not occur. And unless an egg ripens, there will be no corpus luteum to release progesterone—the first hormone to diminish. Despite the fact that the pituitary puts out increased amounts of FSH and LH, the ovaries become less responsive and their production of estrogen eventually ceases.

Menopause occurs on average between the ages of forty-eight and fifty-two, although some women stop menstruating in their late thirties. Regardless of age, women typically experience four to six years when hormone levels progressively decline before menstruation ends, known as perimenopause. Perimenopause is characterized by sharp fluctuations in levels of progesterone. Estrogen levels diminish slowly, but if no egg ripens in a given cycle, progesterone drops abruptly. This causes fluctuations in cycle length, bouts of intermittent bleeding, and varying amounts of blood loss with menstruation. Typically, periods are closer together and much heavier than before; bleeding for a week to ten days is not unusual.

Problems can develop if bleeding is more frequent, or if cumulative blood loss becomes excessive. Sometimes a D&C is recommended to rule out uterine cancer. Fibroids and polyps may also be implicated, but in the vast majority of cases, the problem is simply that progesterone levels are not high enough to maintain the uterine lining. Changes in diet and lifestyle, along with herbal remedies, may offer some relief. Studies show that deficiencies of iron, vitamin C, and bioflavonoids can exacerbate heavy bleeding, as can smoking, stress, and excessive intake of alcohol.

Some women have no trouble with progesterone decrease and simply notice that their periods come less often and are lighter than before. They may be troubled by decreasing estrogen, though, correlated to side effects of hot flashes, mood swings, night sweats, and vaginal changes. Again, nutritional and/or herbal remedies may help (see specific sections on each of these symptoms later in the chapter).

When a woman has stopped menstruating for a full year, her menopause is complete. We then honor her with the title Woman of the Thirteenth Moon. This is the classic time for a menopause celebration or Croning Rite (see boxed section, page 186).

The age at which menopause occurs is somewhat hereditary; if your mother or sisters were later or earlier than average, you are likely to follow suit. Women in industrialized countries are, however, experiencing menopause later and later. The average is now age fifty-one; at the turn of the century it was forty-six. Considering that life expectancy then was little more than fifty years, and it is easy to see the basis of the belief that menopause marks the beginning of the end. But a woman today can expect to live an average of seventy-eight years, thus finishing menopause with nearly a third of her life still ahead of her.

What will this last third of her life be like? Is she doomed, as the media would have us believe, to be shriveled and sexless—a doddery "senior citizen"? This depends largely on how well she takes care of herself physically, and on how she defines herself both personally and socially. But first, she must find a way to make it through "the change."

Male authorities on the subject have been little more than harbingers of doom. Robert A. Wilson, author of *Feminine Forever* and staunch advocate of hormone replacement therapy (HRT), describes menopause as "the loss of womanhood and the loss of good health," claiming that "chemical imbalances" result in castration and a state of "living decay."[1] David Reuben, author of *Everything You Always Wanted to Know About Sex but Were Afraid to Ask*, expresses a similar, antiquated view of menopause as the end for women: "Having outlived their ovaries, they may have outlived their usefulness as human beings. The remaining years may just be marking time until they follow their glands into oblivion."[2]

But women experts have other opinions. Sheila Kitzinger views menopausal changes as those by which "a new balance is found, one which is natural and right for an older woman," through a process she likens to adolescence. She is quick to point out that although estrogen and progesterone diminish, they are effectively counterbalanced by increasing testosterone.[3] Susan Lark, author of *The Menopause Self-Help Book*, notes that because women tend to pay better attention to their health in menopause than ever before, these years can be a time of unprecedented "vigor and vitality."[4] Or, as author Susan Love humorously reminds us, "Your ovaries aren't quitting, they're changing careers, just like the rest of you."[5]

The key is to view menopause as a natural, but major, life transition. It is a period of intense and incontrovertible change, marked by emotional and physical extremes, much like the transition phase of labor, the postpartum period, or the premenstrual phase of the monthly cycle. In all of these, equilibrium is found not by struggling for control, but by surrendering to the change and seeing it through. Coping techniques for PMS, labor, or postpartum can help in menopause, but trust in the process largely determines the ease of its progression.

Much has been said already of how difficult it can be for us to let go this way. Our culture places so great a premium on female constancy that we may deny ourselves opportunities to experience the heights and depths of life as men do, whether by acts of courage or foolishness, creativity or delusion. Nevertheless, a dance of extremes takes place in our flesh, patterned hormonally in our monthly cycle and our Blood Mysteries. Particularly with the latter, we have little choice but to go wild.

Inherent in our wild times is a chance to take stock of ourselves, to assess where we have been and where we have yet to go. Comments like "I no longer love my career" or "I feel alone in my primary relationship" are typical in menopause and hold keys to new directions for the second half of life. Sweeping changes can and should occur at this time. It is foolish not to use the menopause transition for a few radical departures and explorations into the unknown.

Dr. Christiane Northrup and colleague Mona Lisa Schulz are currently at work on a study investigating the roles of FSH and LH during menopause. Much to their surprise, they have found levels of these to be extraordinarily high, approximately a thousand times greater than at any other point in a woman's life! At first glance, this information is confounding—why would the pituitary bother to produce so much FSH and LH at a time when these substances have no apparent function? But preliminary evidence shows FSH and LH to have an entirely different effect in menopausal woman than in women who are still cycling—they serve as neurotransmitters in the right side of the brain, the hemisphere associated with creativity, intuition, and visionary experience.[6]

What a revelation! One of the main reasons I called for a Menopause Council was that I was having an ever-increasing number of intuitive, visionary experiences in my daily life, which I believed must be somehow connected to menopause. That day, I shared that I had gone nine months with no period, but when I unexpectedly bled again it was as if a curtain fell in front of my eyes—the exquisite visionary dimension I had been exploring just slipped away. Northrup's and Schulz's research makes clear that menopause truly is a time when women can access great wisdom, if only they can trust the process.

Thus any aspect of our past that we have difficulty releasing can make menopausal symptoms worse. In this way, dealing with menopause is similar to coping with PMS. Although some of our premenstrual outbursts are irrational and of little consequence, the intensity of these outbursts often reveals how much we are holding in or holding back. The same is true in menopause. In my research, I've found that menopausal women become almost compulsive in their need to get on with their lives, find new work, start new relationships, or do whatever is necessary to be intimate with their own truth.

Physical Symptoms and Treatment
◎

Some symptoms of menopause are autonomic, due to rapid hormonal fluctuations. These include hot flashes, night sweats, heart palpitations, and itching of the skin. Other effects of menopause include vaginal dryness, bladder dysfunction, joint pain, osteoporosis, muscular weakness, wrinkling of the skin, thinning of the hair, weight gain, bloating, and headache. Emotional reactions include moodiness and irritability, insomnia, forgetfulness, and changes in sexual desire. Guidelines for coping with these symptoms fall more or less into one of two camps: obliteration of symptoms through hormonal control, or cooperation with the process via health-enhancing natural practices.

Remember that HRT was originally developed by physicians. Ignorant and fearful of women's bodies, they perceived menopause, as well as birth and menstruation, as disease conditions requiring medication. To illustrate: one of my students recounted that her mother, in labor and at the height of transition, called her doctor a "goddamn son-of-a-bitch" and was sedated without her consent.

Certainly in our culture, men are entirely unprepared to deal with women's biological transitions, particularly when at full throttle, and have thus sought ways to dominate and control women at these critical junctures. Medication is a powerful way to do this. This is not to discount the value of hormone replacement in certain circumstances, but the routine use of hormones to address common complaints of menopause is just as bad as drugging the body in childbirth or obliterating premenstrual symptoms with sedatives.

Author Joan Borysenko comments wryly in one of her lectures that our solution for women's "irrational" behavior is to put them on oral contraceptives at menarche, take them off long enough for childbearing, medicate them for birth, get them back on oral contraceptives until menopause, then start HRT. How would it be, she wonders, if we had a medication for men, "test-away," that could similarly be started at adolescence, stopped briefly for child siring, then continued on through old age? Think how calm and compliant men would be, she muses—no wild drinking, crazy driving, fights, and so on.[7]

What made HRT attractive to women in the first place? When HRT was first developed, it was touted as the only way menopausal women might stay youthful. It was marketed as a panacea for sleeplessness, depression, loss of interest in sex, dry skin and hair, fatigue—in other words, all the undesired effects of aging.

But now the data are in, and the benefits of HRT appear dubious, at best. Even though estrogen may help reduce hot flashes, vaginal changes, and wrinkling of the skin, synthetic forms have serious side effects and contraindications, particularly if taken without progesterone. If synthetic estrogen (ERT) is used exclusively for six or more years, breast cancer rates increase four times, and the risk of uterine cancer is increased ten times. ERT also increases the risk of gall bladder disease, thrombosis, phlebitis, headaches, and depression, and is contraindicated for anyone suffering from liver disease, sickle cell anemia, gall stones, diabetes, or abnormal vaginal bleeding.[8]

Although physicians are increasingly aware of this information and seek to combine estrogen with progesterone as much as possible, it is crucial that any woman on HRT know the signs of estrogen overdose, as each of us has our own level of tolerance. These signs include water retention, folic acid anemia, bloating, nausea, and breast tenderness. Signs of progesterone excess include increased susceptibility to vaginal yeast and other infections, fatigue, and hirsutism (excess body and facial hair).

What about the supposed benefits of HRT in terms of decreased susceptibility to heart disease and osteoporosis? Regarding the latter, please see the forthcoming section on this topic. As for heart disease, a sixteen-year study of forty thousand postmenopausal nurses conducted by Francine Grodstein at Brigham and Women's Hospital in Boston showed that if women do not already have risk factors, HRT is not particularly helpful in terms of prevention.[9] Northrup maintains that increased insulin resistance, present in 50 to 75 percent of women, plays a much more significant role in the development of heart disease. A 1977 study published in the *American Journal of Clinical Nutrition* showed that a high-carbohydrate, excessively low-fat diet put women at risk, deleteriously affecting lipid and insulin levels in the body.[10]

Sedatives and tranquilizers are also commonly prescribed for menopausal women and are sometimes added to the hormonal formula. Since depression is a known side effect of HRT, this seems to make sense. On the other hand, Rosetta Reitz, author of *Menopause: A Positive Approach*, believes tranquilizers are generally prescribed to menopausal women to keep them out of sight and out of mind. "Do you know what would happen if all the women between 40 and 55 started making demands?" she queries. "My adrenaline begins to burst forth at the excitement of the idea." Other drawbacks to tranquilizer use include chemical dependency and the interruption of REM sleep, which is necessary for dreaming.

Tranquilizer use seems misguided, at best, as most studies show menopausal women to be no more inherently depressed than women at other stages of life. Depression associated with HRT is most likely due to a lack of testosterone, which is now being added to some formulas. Without this, libido is often reduced and moods become flat, monotone (much as is true of women on the Pill). Psychologist Barbara Sherwin of McGill University in Montreal demonstrated this in her research on women in their forties who experienced early menopause due to hysterectomy. Compared to women taking estrogen and progesterone only, those whose formulas included testosterone had more intense sexual desires and fantasies, were more easily aroused, and had orgasms more frequently. They also had higher energy levels and a greater sense of well-being.

Herbs such as nettle stimulate the adrenals to produce adequate testosterone, as can supplemental use of DHEA. Red raspberry leaf and hawthorn berry teas invigorate the system and can help alleviate depression, as can St. John's wort.

Although testosterone dips naturally in menopause, it later returns to previous levels and continues to rise steadily as we age. Experiencing decreased levels of testosterone in menopause can be distressing but may serve to refocus us on larger issues in our lives. This account serves to illustrate:

> I've pretty well completed my menopause. I'm begin-
> ning to get my energy back, and I'm not feeling the childlike
> things I felt earlier in my passage. The emotional swings
> were very much like adolescence—I would feel things
> explosively, and tears came very easily. For me, this was all
> part of seeing my attachment to my body, and learning just
> what my body is and isn't. For instance, my libido went way
> down, and I've always had a very strong sex drive—it was just
> like falling off a cliff. I had sworn that I would be vibrantly
> sexual till my dying day, and when I discovered how much
> of that urge was really physiological and driven by
> hormones, I felt a little bit of . . . almost embarrassment at
> my presumption, thinking I knew myself and realizing that
> what I had identified as self was so much physical. At that

point, a lot of things just started falling away, my attachment to relationship and the feeling of protection I'd had by having another person around. I began to see my strength as coming from my own centeredness, centeredness in Spirit.[11]

As we look more closely at specific menopausal symptoms and their potential effect on sexuality, we will consider the risks and benefits of HRT alongside those of herbs, supplements, and dietary changes. (For more detailed information, see the charts on pages 189 and 190.)

Hot Flashes

Three out of four women experience hot flashes, the most common menopausal symptom. Hot flashes are the only symptom considered to be universal, occurring among women almost everywhere in the world. During a hot flash, there is a rush of heat to the chest, neck, and face, or sometimes throughout the body. This can happen anytime, anywhere. The skin reddens, temperature increases, and breathing becomes shallow. There may also be an itching sensation. As the heat passes, women often find themselves drenched in sweat and may then feel chilly and drained. These episodes may or may not be noticed by others; regardless, women are often disoriented or embarrassed by them.

Physically, hot flashes result from vasomotor instability originating in the temperature-regulating center of the hypothalamus. Some women are so susceptible that even subtle temperature changes caused by exercise, stress, sexual arousal, and cold or hot room environments can trigger hot flashes. Some note a strong correlation between drinking caffeinated beverages or alcohol and increased incidence of hot flashes. Large doses of niacin (vitamin B6) and certain drugs, such as those used to treat hypertension, are also implicated. Emotional upsets can trigger hot flashes, too.

Hot flashes are linked to decreasing estrogen and also to high levels of LH common in menopause. The precise mechanism of their occurrence remains unknown. Some women never experience hot flashes; others have them three times a day or more. Many experience them only at night. The hot flashes and night sweats of menopause are very much like those experienced postpartum, which are likewise due to marked hormonal fluctuations. Hot flashes usually persist no more than five years; most women have them for several months only.

Commonsense measures include layering clothing so that certain items can be shed quickly, keeping a spray bottle by the bed, in the car, and at the office, having a change of sheets or towels by the bed, and using a small electric fan when feasible. Although increased estrogen (whether by HRT or natural alternative) can control hot flashes, they come right back when treatment is stopped. Tincture of motherwort, twenty drops under the tongue, is reputed to be one of the best natural remedies. Tincture of black cohosh works well, too. Soy products are also extremely effective; soy is an excellent source of plant-based phyto-estrogens, which are readily absorbed without negative side effects. Bioflavonoids added to the diet or taken supplementally help, too. Homeopathic remedies may also be useful, lachesis in particular. For more information on this and other therapies, see *Menopausal Years: The Wise Woman Way*, by Susun Weed. This is a comprehensive and inspiring book—one of my favorites.[12]

Apart from the nuisance, some women feel hot flashes provide an opportunity to change their perspective. Many of my clients speak in terms of surrendering to their flashes and feeling stimulated, illuminated. Some even say that hot flashes trigger intuitive insights and revelations. Barbara Raskin, author of the book *Hot Flashes*, describes these messages as "urgent communiqués from the interior of a vast, dark continent . . . fast-breaking news items from my heart of darkness."[13] The element of darkness is strongly tied to woman in her Crone aspect: she weaves the web of life and reaps whatever has outlived its usefulness. Hot flashes provide a metaphysical opportunity to connect with the shadow side of our nature and use it to let go of whatever we don't need in life anymore.

Women also find that the better they get to know themselves in menopause, the more likely they are to know when a hot flash is coming. Sometimes a revelation precedes the flash and may thus serve as a signal to take off a sweater or turn on the fan. At the most basic level, hot flashes result from overload of the endocrine system, which is busy adjusting multiple physiological functions to match changed levels of estrogen and progesterone. Overload equals altered state, and that is exactly what hot flashes represent or intimate.

Kitzinger likens the process of coping with hot flashes to that of coping with labor contractions. She recommends slowing down and opening up, breathing from low in the body, down in the pelvis. This can change the experience from upsetting to erotic, bringing a rosy glow to a woman's face and softening her demeanor. We can use hot flashes to experience heightened awareness in a variety of ways, depending on how we focus our attention.

Vaginal and Pelvic Changes

In menopause, vaginal tissues may thin and become easily damaged. There may be some lack of lubrication as well, caused by a reduction of transvaginal electropotential—that is, the mechanism by which water and electrolytes are conveyed across vaginal tissues. None of this affects the libido, but it can certainly influence sex itself.

These changes occur because estrogen levels are diminished, rendering the vagina more alkaline than usual and hence more vulnerable to infection. Decreased estrogen can also lead to reduced vaginal and pelvic circulation, implicating the bladder and accounting for the increased incidence of urinary tract infections.

Of all the symptoms of menopause for which estrogen therapy is suggested, vaginal dryness is the one for which it is most widely used.

Estrogen is readily absorbed by vaginal tissues, and a single course of cream applied by plunger can sometimes turn things around significantly. Lubricating jelly will still be necessary on occasion, or vitamin E might be used alternatively. Seminal fluid has a positive effect on vaginal tissues, as does evening primrose oil; both contain prostaglandins, which soften and condition. And orgasm itself is most beneficial: it stimulates circulation and the release of natural lubrication. According to Rosetta Reitz, intercourse and masturbation on a regular basis make vaginal and pelvic changes at menopause "hardly noticeable." One study showed that weekly intercourse so increased women's estrogen levels that many of these common complaints were eliminated.[14]

As already discussed, continued use of estrogen alone carries significant health risks; therefore, natural alternatives should be tried and used whenever possible. Possibly the most popular of these are the topical application of natural estrogen creams and the addition of soy products to the diet: both are high in phyto-estrogens. Vitamin E, at least 600 IU taken daily, has also proven to be beneficial. Bioflavonoids are important, too; take approximately 800 mg daily, or eat more citrus fruit (especially the inner rind) and buckwheat. Herbal teas of licorice root and black cohosh root also help stimulate estrogen production.

For urinary tract problems, herbs like goldenseal and uva ursi (bearberry) are classic. Goldenseal contains berberine, which has antibiotic affects, and uva ursi has arbutin, a diuretic and anti-infective agent. The two can be combined and simmered slowly to make a tea or may be taken as tincture. See the chart on page 189 for additional ideas.

Osteoporosis

The term *osteoporosis* refers to loss of bone mass, and although it occurs in men, it is more common among women in our culture.

Estrogen plays a critical role in maintaining the structure and calcification of bone, so the decline in this hormone at menopause is thought to precipitate the condition. But there are other factors involved. Genetic predisposition figures strongly in osteoporosis, as does a diet high in salt, animal protein, caffeine, alcohol, or carbonated drinks (high levels of phosphorus directly decrease bone mass). Some authorities feel that inadequate intake of vitamin D may be a primary factor, particularly as exposure to sunlight is increasingly discouraged. This is corroborated by cross-cultural studies showing that osteoporosis is far from universal in menopausal women. Some populations show no osteoporosis in women at any age, while in others both men and women are affected, even prior to midlife. The incidence is definitely higher in industrialized countries, among women who smoke, have a Northern European background, are sedentary, or regularly use drugs such as steroids, diuretics, aluminum-containing antacids, thyroid supplements, and anticonvulsants.

The effects of osteoporosis are worse than the condition itself. The spine tends to compress and curve, and certain bones, particularly the hips, are highly susceptible to fracture. Such injuries usually occur later in life, around ages seventy to eighty. But 30 percent of women thus affected die of complications, and many more suffer chronic disability.

It seems obvious that diet and lifestyle are major factors in osteoporosis. What are some of the ways we can prevent this condition from developing? First, we must stop worrying about the extra five or ten pounds typically gained at menopause and start focusing more on nutrition (ideally, long before menopause occurs). There is evidence that our ability to absorb calcium from dairy products decreases with age, so we must find other sources. Calcium citrate, found almost exclusively in products like orange juice with added calcium, is much more readily absorbed than is calcium lactate. Enriched soy products are also good sources of calcium, as are dark leafy green vegetables and seeds, especially sesame.

Calcium is, however, just one of many nutrients essential to good health. An optimal diet for menopause should consist of plenty of green and yellow vegetables, legumes, fresh fruits in season, complex carbohydrates, nuts and seeds, and minimal amounts of animal protein except for fish, which is an excellent source of the omega fatty acids. Particularly important are trace minerals, but these are often leached from the soil by commercial farming methods. Organic fruits and vegetables are as much as five times higher in nutritional value than their commercial counterparts. It is definitely worth finding a store that stocks organic produce.[15] See the box on page 190 for more details on nutrition in menopause.

Supplements can also help increase or maintain bone density. Calcium, magnesium, boron, vitamin C, and vitamin D all play crucial roles in preventing osteoporosis. Natural progesterone cream also seems to have a positive effect.

Our busy and erratic lifestyle also has negative effects on our health. Most of us spend way too much time indoors, sitting at a desk or doing housework that keeps us just this side of aerobic, chronically tense with the pressure of having so many things to do. This is diametrically opposed to what we truly need: good food, regular exercise, and daily relaxation in complementary measure. In fact, next to getting enough calcium in the diet, the single most important way to avoid osteoporosis is with weight-bearing exercise—basically, any upright activity such as walking, dancing, bicycling, climbing stairs, or lifting light weights. As women, we are especially apt to defer to the needs of others and may thus deprive ourselves of these health-promoting necessities. Eventually, and sometimes with surprising swiftness, this can catch up with us.

* * *

In her bestseller *The Silent Passage*, Gail Sheehy portrays common complaints of menopause as universally disruptive and virtually incapacitating. Yet the data show that many women sail through menopause with little trouble. For others, fear may exacerbate initial symptoms just enough to drive them to seek hormone replacement, much as fear in labor makes contractions infinitely harder to handle and leads women to ask for drugs. Once a woman is on this track, it can be tricky to get off.

It's a good idea to ask your mother or older sisters what menopause was like for them, because patterns and severity of symptoms tend to be somewhat hereditary. Even more important are the coping mechanisms your female relations used: what worked and what didn't. I was relieved when my mother told me that menopause had been a breeze for her; she had occasional hot flashes at night and that was about it. But if your family history is not so rosy, don't panic. Get the complete picture, making sure to factor in the effects of medical interventions and lifestyle before jumping to any conclusions.

Sex During Menopause
◎

What is sex like at this time? Reports range wildly, from plain disinterest to blooming desire. Decreased testosterone levels, although temporary, may put a damper on passion, but so can emotional revelations. From Marjorie:

> Looking back, I think my moodiness had a lot to do with
> it. I never really let go of wanting to have a second child,
> even though the years went by and nothing happened. Then
> menopause put an end to that dream, and I cried and raged
> at my husband, to the point that he called the doctor for

sedatives! I tried estrogen for a while but just got more depressed. I wanted absolutely nothing to do with Blake . . . I acted as though it was all his fault. And I really did blame him—when I wanted kids early in our marriage, he wasn't ready, and then we had to wait so long for our son. Anyway, my hot flashes were awful, they happened to me everywhere and often made me cry. Sometimes I'd come home and scream in the closet, when no one was around.

We didn't have sex, except once in a while when I felt I could stomach it, like once a month or so. After it [menopause] was all over, though, I got my drive back all right . . . I only wish my husband had. Things are different between us now . . . I guess we'll never be the same.

Quite the opposite experience, from Geri:

Menopause was liberation for me. I didn't expect it, but so it was. No more worries about birth control—after four children, free at last! By then, the youngest was almost full grown. I took classes at the local college, art and creative writing. I felt so good to finally be able to go after my dreams. And sex, well, we reached new heights with it. My drive became more intense, my confidence increased, my husband loved it! He began to take more time with me, feeding my senses and enjoying my rhythms. We were really on a par.

Geri's story is actually a bit more postmenopausal. Here is Elaine's tale, from deep in the thick of it:

I welcomed menopause; I wasn't afraid because I'd learned to trust my body over the years and felt ready for whatever it had in store for me. The intensity of the hot flashes threw me at first, but I began to see them as a sort of energy release. When I looked at menopause as a transition to my wiser, seasoned self, I decided that with every flash, I'd let something go—some obligation to someone else's priorities, some outdated idea of myself, some old wound. It was exhilarating to do this—really a rush! Sometimes I'd flash during intercourse, usually at the beginning of arousal, and I'd use it to boost my passion. My partner had no complaints. He didn't always know what was up, but sex often took the edge off my sharpness. Menopausal women are so powerful—I think men can be intimated by the change. For us, sex was the bridge.

Diane says this of her experience with Elsa:

I was in menopause before my partner, by about a year or so. We both experienced hot flashes for a while, although hers were usually more intense. It was fun, and really wonderful for both of us to have the support and understanding. Minor inconveniences some women speak of, like vaginal dryness—applying oils to each other just became part of our sexual pleasure. But the dimension menopause opened for us was the big surprise . . . we had always been telepathic to some extent, but now we could read each other with ease.

Last, a classically mixed response:

I grieved during menopause—I hate to admit it, because I consider myself a liberated woman—but I was deeply afraid of growing old, of losing my looks. This affected my self-confidence and desire for sex. I was afraid I'd lose my husband, so I shut down in bed—I was scared of being vulnerable. When my hot flashes were the most intense we stopped making love for a while, I guess for about three months or so. My vagina felt different too, drier and very tender. In retrospect, I think I was testing my husband, and lo and behold, after it was all over, he was still there. Then my desire skyrocketed, and I took hold of the situation.

Thus far, we've considered menopause only as a natural phenomenon. When it is surgically induced, as by hysterectomy, the experience is very different. Instead of a gradual decline in hormonal levels, a woman experiences abrupt withdrawal—her system is thrown into shock.

Hysterectomy is the second most common major surgical procedure in the United States. In 1991, 544,000 American women had hysterectomies; it is estimated that there will be 824,000 hysterectomies in the year 2005. This is an extremely high rate—up to four times higher than that of other industrialized nations.[16] The average age of a woman undergoing hysterectomy is 42.7 years. A majority of gynecologists actually believe that women beyond their childbearing prime are safer without their reproductive organs—"the uterus is for growing babies or for growing cancer."[17] This view utterly discounts the physical difficulties and emotional trauma women typically experience when the menopause transition occurs so abruptly. Even when there are clear indications for surgery, loss of her reproductive organs can cause a woman to sink into depression and undergo a classic process of grieving.

There are four main indications for hysterectomy: (1) cancer of the reproductive organs; (2) severe infection of the fallopian tubes, uterus, or ovaries that cannot be controlled; (3) extremely large fibroid tumors; and (4) uncontrollable uterine bleeding unresponsive to D&C or any other remedy. Yet these conditions account for only

12 percent of all hysterectomies—indicating that the majority are probably unnecessary.

When hysterectomy is recommended for fibroids or uterine bleeding, the ovaries do not have to be removed, particularly if the woman is over forty, when her risk of ovarian cancer drops to 1 percent. Subtotal hysterectomy, whereby the ovaries or some part thereof are saved, is always best because even a small portion of a single ovary can continue hormonal production. If the difficulty is fibroids alone, a myomectomy may permit surgical removal of the fibroid while saving the uterus. Although fibroid tissue tends to grow back, myomectomy is the best solution for the woman whose fibroid has grown cumbersome (they can reach a weight of one hundred pounds) and who still desires children.

Sex for the woman who has undergone complete hysterectomy is apt to be distressing both physically and emotionally. Annette recalls, "I felt empty, like I had nothing to offer anymore. My muscles were all shot and soft—my vagina was foreign territory to me and I wasn't sure I wanted to get to know it again. Having to face the fact that I'd never have a child and would never give birth was unspeakably painful to me, and stole the magic from sex and my body for a very long time." Another woman reports, "The inside of me felt all stopped up and rigid—like a dead-end, literally. I had periodic bleeding at first, which was normal, they said. Even though it was scary, I actually welcomed it—at least something was coming out of me! When I bled, I found that I could cry. After it stopped, I turned my sadness inward until I healed."

On the other side, here's an account from Mandy: "I had suffered so tremendously with endometriosis and recurrent uterine infection that the decision for hysterectomy came as a relief. I wasn't sure I wanted kids anyway, and now the matter was settled. But I noticed a funny thing: for months after the surgery, I still felt a rhythm, a ghost cycle I guess. I didn't know how much that rhythm had become a part of me, wracked with pain as I was."

Some women notice a change in orgasms after hysterectomy. The deep contractions felt in the uterus, or the stimulation of the cervix that some women find so pleasurable, are no longer part of the experience. This sort of sexual crisis necessitates refocusing and reconditioning oneself (and one's partner) to find satisfaction in other pleasure centers.

The symptoms of surgically induced menopause are usually so extreme as to necessitate HRT, at least for a while. Many women try to taper their formula down to a minimal level by their late forties and discontinue in their fifties. Others choose to stay on HRT indefinitely.

Brooke Medicine Eagle, a Native American authority on women's health issues, speaks frequently on the meaning of surgical menopause. She speculates that hysterectomy in the childbearing years may afford certain women the opportunity to assume mature leadership roles traditionally held by their elders, due to our deficit in women's wisdom and the urgent need for its resurgence. In her tradition, whenever and however menopause occurs, it marks a time when a woman retains her precious menstrual fluid or "wise blood" for increased awareness and greater wisdom. Postmenopausal women of the Grandmother Lodge are thus accorded the deepest respect and the highest honor.[18]

Celebrating "the Change"

In Native American and many other indigenous cultures, women at menopause are honored by rites that help them celebrate the event and more deeply appreciate its meaning. However, menopause in our culture is often accompanied by feelings of sadness and uncertainty. What sort of ritual might we employ to help us acknowledge these feelings, while at the same time exploring the great potential of this transition?

Most menopause rituals naturally incorporate practices for letting go of the past and welcoming new responsibilities. For example, women may gather around a fire (or a symbolic candle) and take turns, one by one, giving up some fear, resentment, or self-limiting belief to be consumed by the flame. If the fire is large enough, each woman can throw in a token of her surrender—a piece of wood, paper, cloth, or other symbolic item.

As each woman takes her turn, she speaks of her deepest lesson in life, and of that which she still intends to accomplish. Members of the group can acknowledge what she has said and charge her with the responsibility of serving as a caretaker of life via her special gifts and vision. It's best to have women of all ages present at a menopause rite: the Crones, Matriarchs, Mothers, and Maidens.

In essence, the transition to Cronehood signifies a time when women transmute their personal pursuits and the demands of child-bearing to become "keepers of the law." Their role shifts from nurturing their immediate families to caring for humanity. Their seasoned sense of justice and their peacekeeping abilities are now available to society. The word *Crone* is actually similar in derivation to *crown*, signifying leadership. Even the word *hag*, which has such a derogatory meaning in our culture, comes from the Greek *hagia*, meaning "a holy one."[19]

In yet another ritual, everyone gathers around a large bowl or pot of water. Each has a cup, and moving clockwise, each takes a turn to dip and drink, saying, "I accept the wisdom of ages past." The Crones then form an inner circle. One begins by saying what she has learned in life, what wisdom she still seeks, or what she must do to complete her life's mission. As she finishes, the Crone to her right reminds her, "Take from the wisdom of the ages the means to fulfill your destiny," or "Shed the skin that has become too tight for you and be born anew."[20] Each takes a turn, moving around the circle until all have spoken.

When the Crones are done, the outer circle of women repeats the process. As each finishes speaking, the Crones respond in turn by repeating the one of the blessings given above.

Although these rituals work best in groups, the same acts of letting go of the past, naming life lessons, and identifying the keys to one's future may also be done in solitude. Use a candle, water, or both, and be sure to give voice to your thoughts: the power of the spoken word is great. Also see the boxed section below for cross-cultural Croning customs.

The Croning Rite

Ancient Queen of Wisdom
Hecate, Cerridwyn
Old One—Come to Us!

This rite of passage is observed when a woman has completed menopause, with no menstruation for a full year. The post-menopausal stage heralds the start of a new life phase, when she is to be venerated for her life experience. It is a time of celebration. Or, if a woman has undergone premature menopause due to surgical or chemical intervention, she may have her croning ritual whenever she wants.

Menopause honoring still occurs in non-industrial societies, but these rites are increasingly contaminated by patriarchal feelings of shame and disgust. This is why it is so important to recreate these rites, lest they be obliterated.

In the Seneca tradition, a woman entering perimenopause speaks with the Grandmothers of her tribe and chooses a subject to teach the young women of her community. Possible subjects include the spirituality of dreams, animals, trees, or food. Or she may choose to address the challenges of maturation for women and children. After teaching for a year, she becomes a Grandmother and is revered as a wise one. When her menopause is finally complete, she is accorded the further honor of being allowed to select the chiefs of her tribe.

Older women of some Jewish congregations mark the transition from mother to elder authority by changing their names. In similar fashion, Native American women are often given new names at menopause by their chief.

The menopause rite is designed around a standard format. The woman's female friends and relations gather to decorate the room, using evergreens, which signify immortality, or other boughs of winter classically representing the Crone. The circle may then be smudged, and the four directions or four faces of the Goddess called in, particularly Hecate of the North, who represents the crossroads of life and immortality. The ceremony can begin by weaving a "Mother Line": as participants pass a candle or ceremonial object around the circle, each speaks her name and that of her mother, grandmother and great-grandmother, going back in her female lineage as far as she can remember. "I am Susan, daughter of Caroline, granddaughter of Rose, great-granddaughter of Violet."

The body of the rite can take various forms. I recall the rite we held for a Crone midwife who was retiring from active practice. Each midwife in attendance shared a memory of working with her, and as they told their stories they wove red, white, and black yarn, along with some special trinket, into a "story belt." Some of the stories were hilarious, but the result was a poignant, ceremonial object of inestimable value. Or, the women in the circle can take turns telling the Crone what it has meant to have her as a friend, or ask her an important personal question in hopes that, with her newfound authority, she will provide wise counsel. To close, a pomegranate is given to her and she is to ingest as many seeds as years she has lived, with as many blessings for continued fruitfulness in the years to come.

The Crone can conclude her rite privately, going off to a three-way crossroads only she knows, where she offers food and prayer to Hecate:

"I have traveled the road from my mother's breast to Cronehood. Thank you, Hecate, for the good seasons past and the good seasons yet to come."[21]

It is best to do this particular part of the ritual at the dark moon or earliest crescent, as this lunar phase represents regeneration, a time of new beginnings. The Crone must make her offering and not look back, to signify letting go of regrets while trusting what is yet to come. An aspect of seclusion is found in numerous other rites, and is symbolic of rebirth. Meanwhile, her friends feast and make merry and prepare to welcome her return. With love and laughter, they share food, stories, songs, vision.

"Nascent rites can be enlarged and formalized. What is required is a small community of family and friends, some symbolic and traditional sources of inspiration, a clear formulation of the change involved and its significance—and courage."[22]

Reprinted from *The Women's Wheel of Life: Thirteen Archetypes of Woman at Her Fullest Power*, by Elizabeth Davis and Carol Leonard

Symptoms in Menopause and
Their Treatment

◉

	Nutritional Supplements	**Natural Sources**
Excess bleeding	Vitamin A 5,000 IU	Hawthorn berry
		Vitex
	Vitamin C 1,000 mg	Dandelion root
	Iron 30 mg	Shepherd's purse
	Bioflavonoids 800 mg	Black haw
		False unicorn
		Sarsaparilla
		Wild yam root
Hot flashes	Vitamin E 800 IU	Motherwort
	Bioflavonoids 800 mg	Dong quai
		Black cohosh
		Fennel
		Pomegranate
Vaginal changes	Vitamin E 800 IU	Motherwort
	Bioflavonoids 800 mg	Saw palmetto berries
	Evening primrose oil	Comfrey ointment
	Linseed oil	
Urinary tract problems	Vitamin C 1,000–1,500 mg	Uva ursi
		Nettle
		Goldenseal
		Black currant
		Yarrow
Osteoporosis	Vitamin D 5,000 IU	Oat straw
	Calcium citrate 1,500 mg	Nettle
	Folic acid 800 mcg	Comfrey root
	Zinc 20 mg	Horsetail
	Magnesium 500 mg	

	Nutritional Supplements	Natural Sources
Nervous irritability	Vitamin B complex 50 mg	Passionflower
	Vitamin C 1,000 mg	Valerian root
	Bioflavonoids 800 mg	Hops
		Catnip
Fatigue, depression	Vitamin B complex 50 mg	Ginger
	Vitamin C 1,000 mg	Cayenne pepper
	Magnesium 500 mg	Oat straw
	Potassium aspartate 100 mg	Blessed thistle

Nutrition in Menopause

Good nutrition is of utmost importance during menopause. As we age, the digestive tract produces fewer enzymes and less hydrochloric acid. Yet many menopausal problems and complaints can be minimized or alleviated by eating the right foods.

Whole Grains

Whole grains include whole corn and wheat, unhulled barley, oats, rye, millet, buckwheat, brown rice, and wild rice. They stabilize blood-sugar levels and reduce sugar cravings. They also help to prevent diabetes and may also protect against cancer of the colon because they are high in fiber. Eat freely of these, and try for some variety each week. Raw wheat germ is a good source of vitamin E, helpful for vaginal dryness and other low estrogen symptoms.

Legumes

Legumes are the peas and beans, such as lentils, kidney beans, black beans, chickpeas, pinto beans, white beans, and split peas. All are high in protein and fiber and digest slowly, making them especially appropriate for older women. Problems with gas can be alleviated by slow and thorough cooking, or by eating small amounts.

Vegetables

Vegetables provide a full range of vitamins and minerals. The dark green, orange, and red varieties are high in vitamin A, which has been shown to protect against cancer of the breast and cervix, as well as immunological disease. Vitamin C has similar benefits, and it additionally helps to prevent excessive bleeding at menopause if combined with iron and bioflavonoids. Good sources of vitamin C include peppers, potatoes, peas, tomatoes, broccoli, cabbage, parsley, and kale. Vegetables also provide important minerals such as calcium, magnesium, iron, zinc, copper, and trace elements if grown organically. Onions and garlic help lower serum cholesterol, reducing the risk of strokes and heart attacks. Seaweeds such as kelp and nori are high in iodine, which promotes healthy thyroid function.

Fruits

Fruits also provide a wide range of vitamins and minerals. They are especially rich in potassium, which serves to regulate blood pressure. Potassium also helps prevent the fatigue commonly associated with menopause. Especially good sources are bananas, berries, melons, grapefruit, peaches, and apricots. High fiber content is yet another bonus of eating fresh fruit, as it helps alleviate constipation. Pineapple and papaya specifically aid digestion by breaking down proteins.

Seeds and Nuts

Seeds and nuts are good sources of protein, but they are very high in fat and calories and thus should be eaten sparingly. Magnesium, potassium, and calcium are quite concentrated in nuts and seeds, particularly almonds, sunflower seeds, pumpkin seeds, and sesame seeds. They digest best if eaten raw, ground into meal or butter.

Fish and Poultry

Red meats are high in fat and hard to digest, and they are often laden with hormones and preservatives. Fish from unpolluted waters and organic poultry are preferred sources of animal protein. Fish is an outstanding source of linoleic acid, which can help with dryness of the hair, skin, and vaginal tissues (this may also be taken supplementally as linseed oil, in liquid or capsule form). Fish is also a good source of the omega fatty acids, known to help prevent neurological problems associated with age, such as Alzheimer's disease.

Foods to Avoid

Salt In excess, salt can exacerbate bloating, high blood pressure, heart disease, and osteoporosis.

Sugar Too much sugar can accelerate diabetes, deplete essential vitamins and minerals, and cause stress, anxiety, and vulnerability to infection.

Caffeine Excess caffeine can cause mood swings, interfere with carbohydrate metabolism, exacerbate hot flashes, and worsen osteoporosis.

Alcohol Alcohol has similar effects to those of caffeine. It also disrupts the liver's ability to metabolize hormones, intensifying menopausal complaints.

Fats Saturated fats, found in dairy products and meats, are especially bad for menopausal women because they are correlated to heart disease, high blood pressure, stroke, and cancer of the ovaries, breasts, and uterus.

Adapted from *The Menopause Self-Help Book* by Susan Lark, M.D. (Berkeley, CA.: Celestial Arts, 1990).

Sex in
Later Years

*It Can Get
Better!*

Just how satisfying a woman's sex life will be once she is past menopause depends largely on how well she retains her self-respect and enthusiasm for living. Against all odds, she must define her continued growth and her newfound authority as valuable, despite society's views to the contrary. So pervasive is the image of older women as used up or outmoded that this task can be difficult indeed. Culturally, we value women primarily for their physical beauty and willingness to serve others. No wonder many women suffer as they age, as their children leave home, and as their family obligations lessen.

One of our finest references for tracking demeaning attitudes toward older women is Barbara Walker's *The Crone*. Walker documents that in pre-Christian societies worldwide, the mythic triumvirate of Virgin, Mother, and Crone reigned supreme. Christian mythology virtually eradicated the Crone, retaining only the more benign and readily controlled Maiden and Mother figures.[1]

What made the Crone so threatening? In the Hindu tradition, she was known as Kali the Destroyer—not that she was maliciously violent or spiteful, but she did possess fierce instincts to terminate anything that had exhausted its usefulness so that it might be transformed to something new. Accordingly, her power was tremendous. In myth after myth, the Crone persona proved stronger than any god. As the Teutonic Elli, she conquered Thor, the god of strength. As the Celtic Morgan Le Fay (or Morgan of the Fates), she had the power to humble and tame all men. As the Greek Atropos the Cutter, she snipped the thread of every life.

The aspect of the Crone most frightening to men of any age is her power to reject, to refuse to care for their personal concerns to the exclusion of her care for society at large. Women's power to say no, to see and serve a higher moral code or natural law, is what men have sought so persistently and desperately to obliterate. Not only were midwives prime targets of the Inquisition, old women were, too, particularly if they held their own property and were financially independent.[2]

It is a little-known fact that our U.S. Constitution is a nearly perfect copy of the Iroquois model of leadership—with which Thomas Jefferson was most impressed—except for one critical omission. We left out the Grandmother Council, the backbone of tribal decision making throughout Native American culture. Imagine how different society might be if the counsel of our female elders was sought on all major environmental, economic, or political issues. Doubtless, the Grandmothers' advice would be in frequent opposition to male predilections for war, aggression, domination, and wastefulness, as well as the irrational justification of these.

Fortunately, there are some contemporary cultures that continue to hold elder women in great esteem. In Japan, a woman reaches the highest and most venerated stage of maturity at age sixty-one, an event marked always by ceremony. In certain Native American and South American Indian cultures, postmenopausal women acquire special status and privileges in the community as they transcend menstrual taboos. In China, too, elder woman are venerated and accorded respect.

Beyond honor and veneration, elder women in early matrilineal cultures of the Middle East and Egypt had opportunities to perform society's most important and challenging roles. They dominated the healing arts, working as physicians, surgeons, midwives, and experts on child rearing and sexuality. As scribes, they recorded for both temple and court, maintaining vital records and histories, setting up calendars and official tables of weights and measures, transcribing and editing scriptures, running libraries. They were generally busier in their Crone years than in the childbearing cycle. Mythology reminds us that critical inventions in the fields of medicine, nutrition, and food preparation were made by women in their "years of wisdom."[3]

This last point raises an interesting question. How many years of wisdom did women actually have in these bygone eras? Isn't it true that until quite recently, the average life span for women was barely past menopause?

Contrary to popular belief, there is new evidence that prehistoric women probably survived well past menopause. Anthropologists have struggled to make sense of this from an evolutionary standpoint: What was the point of women living long beyond their reproductive years? Based on their research of a tribe of modern-day hunter-gatherers known as the Hazda, Dr. Kristen Hawkes and colleagues believe that elder women of prehistory made an enormous, quantifiable difference to their kin. Among the Hazda, for example, whenever a mother of young children has another baby and becomes absorbed with breast-feeding, it is only by intervention of an older female relative that the weight (and health) of her other children are maintained:

> When a young woman [of the Hazda tribe] is burdened
> with a suckling infant and cannot fend for her family, she
> turns for support, not to her mate, but to a senior family rela-
> tive—her mother, an aunt, an elder cousin. It is Grandma,
> or Grandma-proxy, who keeps the woman's other children
> in baobab and berries, Grandma who keeps them alive. She
> is not a sentiment, she is a requirement.[4]

On this basis, Hawkes and colleagues developed the Grandmother Hypothesis. They see the extension of life past menopause as a watershed event in our prehistory. For once elder women were available to care for and secure food for the young, the other adults were free to roam and colonize new territories. Quite the opposite was true of primates whose juveniles had to feed themselves; they were confined to feeding grounds where the pickings were easy for young fingers. But with Grandma available to help, humans could migrate to places where securing food required full adult strength and cunning.[5]

Surely this is the most enduring and powerful role of women throughout time, that of Grandmother. Even today, grandmothering makes all the difference to the child of a stressed and busy mother, as well as to the mother herself. The Grandmother keeps the family together. Her nearly invisible role in our culture is one of real influence, in that attitudes, customs, ethical guidelines, and solutions to life's dilemmas are thus passed down through the matrilineal line.

Besides earthly responsibilities, elder women of matrilineal cultures had metaphysical charges too. They facilitated most religious rites and official ceremonies, from birth to death. In terms of the afterlife, it was generally believed that one was taken up in the arms of the Mother, rather than, as by Christian tenets, to the bosom of the Father. In Buddhist and other Tantric traditions, three classes of priestess—*yogini, matri,* and *dakini*—represented the Virgin, Mother, and Crone. Dakini (the Crone) literally means "skywalker"; devoted to the destructive aspect, she prepared the dying for death, worked with bereaved families, and administered last rites. She also knew the way into the spirit realm and could be either fierce or gentle, depending on the dying one's behavior in life and lessons yet to be learned in crossing over.

Similarly, Luisa Francia calls the Crone the "goddess of the crossroads" who can hinder or block one's way, kill, or allow one to pass.[6] Tales and legends from all over the world teach that the path to knowledge or true love inevitably leads through an old woman, a witch, or a woodswoman. She may appear to be so fragile or foolish that no one takes her seriously, and then suddenly she shows her power. In the West, we know her as the trickster Hecate. In Syria, she is the huge-eyed goddess Mari, who searches men's souls. Her Christian adaptation is Aynat, the all-seeing Evil Eye. To a large extent, the ability to look through the veil that hides the future was the province of the Crone, although superstition often led to her being blamed for events she had merely foretold.

Yet another mythic figure symbolizing the power of the Crone is Shakti, an amalgam of queenly strength, intelligence, grace, and sensuality (Shakti is defined as feminine/sexual strength). Across the board, Crone figures possess a strong sexual dimension, which clearly fits with what we know of the postmenopausal increase in testosterone. It's not the sensuality of the Crone that is frightening to men, but the combination of sexual power with emotional discernment and intellectual detachment. The latter is largely due to decreased amounts of estrogen/progesterone, relieving a woman not only of monthly rounds of desire but of emotional dependence on her partner.

Authors Rhonda L. Winn and Niles Newton compiled some fascinating research on sexuality and aging. In most indigenous societies, they found older women to be extremely interested in sex. In 22 percent of these, women became markedly less inhibited with regard to sexual conversation, sexual humor, and sexual gestures as they aged. And in 70 percent of the societies surveyed (including the Loredu of South Africa, the Woges of New Guinea, and the Trobriand and Eastern Islanders), older women frequently had much younger men as sexual partners. Even very old women, described by observers as "toothless and decrepit," were able to obtain young and attractive boys as lovers. Often, older women played the role of sexual initiator and instructor.

In a number of societies surveyed, older women displayed a wide range of sexually suggestive behaviors in public, from making copulatory movements while dancing to grabbing men's genitals or their own, often in a spirit of play. Similarly, they showed great fondness for risqué jokes and anecdotes.[7] Why does this occur? Apart from soaring testosterone levels, the open sexuality of older women is a natural expression of power in cultures where they maintain dominant social roles. It is noteworthy that in societies that frown on sexual activity among the aged, younger individuals tend to view their elders as undesirable or even repulsive.[8]

This has been more or less the case in the United States. According to a Consumers' Union survey entitled "Love, Sex and Aging," some 4,296 respondents concurred that society considered them nonsexual.[9] Only 65 percent of women over seventy were sexually active. A number of these had outlived their husbands and reportedly felt unprepared for the challenge of finding new partners, or were confounded by the threat of sexually transmitted disease. But as the baby boomers age, their characteristic pursuit of self-fulfillment will most likely extend to enduring sexual expression. And as for women outliving men, some predict that we will see increasing acceptance of lesbian coupling as an option for older women (not to mention women in general).

On the other hand, as we live longer, couples will spend an unprecedented number of years together. Rosalie Gilford, sociologist, sums it up this way: "Never in history have the lives of husbands and wives remained interwoven in intact marriages so long as to encounter the constellation of life-changing events that the last stages of the marital career now bring."[10] Unsettling discoveries of differences can certainly arise with time, particularly if the couple has organized itself primarily around child rearing. And hormonally induced role reversal continues to intensify with aging. But if a couple is able to embrace these changes by giving each other space, a more androgynous companionship may ensue.

In bed, interesting possibilities develop. The combination of men's slower arousal time and women's increased aggressiveness can lead to long, drawn-out, even ritualistic (Tantric) lovemaking, with women in the lead. As Charlotte reports:

James and I have been together for forty-three years. We have four grown children and seven grandchildren. I suppose our sex life in the early years was like most others: James came quickly, was a little lacking in touch and timing, and my orgasms were sporadic at best. But I always loved to masturbate, and now, with the standards changing as they are, I find I can talk to him about the intimate details of my body. At first, I think I talked to help cover his embarrassment at slowing down, complimenting him and teaching him at the same time, you might say. But oh, the times we have now! It's hours of pleasure for both of us!

Angelina has a different sort of story:

After I went through "the change" I felt different . . . drier, sometimes, and quite unsure of myself. But I wasn't the only one. Robert took longer to come around, and wanted to spend more time touching than ever before. At first, we were rather confused by all this, but eventually, our affection and companionship deepened, and we felt more alike, more in harmony with one another.

From Suzanne:

The best thing about sex after menopause is not caring anymore . . . sex no longer preoccupies your mind, your time, your body, you're not a victim of your drives. But when you get to it, it's just as good as ever, or even better. Maybe it's more like sex becomes part of everything else in your life. I honestly felt when menopause ended that I was no longer down in the dregs of my hormones, I was above it all, I had this overview all the time, and sex is thoroughly mixed into that.

And from Jeanne:

> I'm almost seventy now, but I can't say that I feel old. Oh, sometimes I have days when I take it a bit slower, but generally, I feel vigorous and self-possessed. I've had my career, and children of whom I'm exceedingly proud—grandchildren, too!
>
> Menopause was upsetting for me because my life was so hectic then, and I think my marriage suffered. But a few years later, something came over me and I felt this strength and confidence in myself, which reached full bloom in the bedroom. I had always liked sex and had orgasms easily, but now, there was another dimension. I'd lift off, in my own thoughts and imagination, and experience a shift in consciousness, almost on a regular basis. You know how it is when you're swept away completely by orgasm, with no idea how you got there? Well, now I seemed to have ready access to those places—freedom to fly, I called it. Really, this was quite the opposite of what I expected sex to be like at this time of my life!

This account ties directly back to the power and authority of the Crone, and it raises the crucial question, How can we realize the full dimensions of Cronehood in our present-day society? Or, to put it in Jeanne's terminology, where do we find the freedom to fly, to traverse the higher realms with ease and confidence?

One way is to act on our natural authority at this stage and seek opportunities to sit in council and employ our wisdom. According to the Native American "law of good relationship," the Grandmothers had the final say in setting right any social or political misdeeds. For example, if a chief was not leading his tribe in such a way that the people had adequate food, water, and shelter, the Grandmothers saw to it that he was replaced. Or, if in times of war a chief instigated animosity to an extent that the tribe's well-being was severely threatened, the Grandmothers might either redirect him or have him removed. Today, women's groups increasingly rally around issues of health care, the environment, education, gun control, and violence, and older women need to let their voices be heard and assume their natural role of leadership in these groups. In this vein, Kitzinger describes postmenopausal women in peasant societies of China and Spain as "political dynamos, wheeling and dealing, plotting and scheming."[11] Form your own elder council or circle, explore the talents, passions, and leadership potential of each woman involved, then get out in the world and make a difference!

On the other hand, there is something of a twist for many postmenopausal women when it comes to taking on additional responsibility. Loss of youthful vigor, loss of children from the home, loss of one's own parents, and ultimately, loss of interest in maintaining "the nest" may lead the elder woman to weed out her possessions and pare her life down to the essentials. Although this nest-dismantling behavior is often miscast as symptomatic of "postmenopausal depression," it is really quite common. Walking away from former entanglements for a simpler way of life makes sense for women at this time.

Another gem of wisdom gleaned from the Menopause Council: when I asked how I might increase my visionary experience, they advised me to (1) do less and (2) be unafraid to hold the big space, especially if it looks like there's nothing in it. Thus, in keeping with the idea of role reversal at menopause, a woman who has played an active role in the world might choose to go into retreat, to travel on her own, or to relocate to a smaller and more suitable nest. Whatever we choose, the need for radical departure from obligatory roles as a means of finding deep intimacy with all of life is the key. It is within this framework that sexual fulfillment may be realized, if we so desire.

Sexual
Abuse and
Dysfunction

Ways to Heal

Why a chapter on abuse in a book on sexual passages? Because most of us have experienced some form of violation, whether emotional, physical, or gynecological, that has negatively affected our sexuality. Sexual dysfunction occurs when we have lost the ability to be sexually self-determined and we have more or less sexual activity than suits us, whether by denial, inhibition, or compulsion. We may, for example, be unable to relate sexually because of unresolved trauma in a relationship, or we may overindulge in sex as an addictive behavior.

We touched only briefly on abuse issues in Chapter 4, in terms of the potential of pregnancy to trigger memories of injuries long forgotten. It is estimated that at least one in four women have been sexually abused, and many do not remember it. How do we dredge from the depths what lies buried? How do we remember abuse?

Workshops on the subject are now widely available. Women who attend may think they are doing so out of simple curiosity; others feel somewhat bewildered as to why they are there until some long-repressed incident comes suddenly into focus. Skeptics say these workshops encourage women to fabricate memories by a process of group hypnosis or induced trance. Nonetheless, there is growing acknowledgment of how commonplace abuse is in our culture and of its devastating effects on our health, self-esteem, and ability to form and sustain healthy relationships. At least women are now encouraged to acknowledge a history of abuse rather than ignore it, as was previously expected.

Sexual and Physical Abuse

A slow but undeniable shift is under way in cultural attitudes regarding abuse. Until quite recently, our criminal justice system showed great reluctance to prosecute abusers, particularly on the basis of children's testimony. Throughout the world, the belief that females are somehow responsible for their own abuse is deeply ingrained. Jurors sometimes still decide that if a girl over the age of seven or so is abused, it is partially because she has behaved or dressed seductively. Women who are raped must often face similar assumptions; they may be grilled as to what they wore or how they behaved when the crime occurred, as though they had played an accessory role.

Rape is an ugly and difficult issue. Once every six minutes in the United States, and once every ninety seconds in South Africa, a woman is raped. As much as possible, we must take measures to protect ourselves—we must be realistic about our vulnerability and avoid situations that might jeopardize us. In the end, even when a case goes to trial and a woman is vindicated, she usually bears scars of her violation that are very difficult to heal.

Date rape is in a class by itself. When a woman is raped by someone she agreed to go out with, it is easier for her to fall victim to guilt and repress the incident. The same is true for the woman raped by her partner or spouse. One way to check into this for yourself is to answer the following questions. Have you ever been made to have sex against your will? Have you ever been forcibly restrained or held down for sex while clearly indicating you wanted to be free? If so, you have indeed been raped.

Questions used to unearth sexual abuse by an acquaintance or relative are more subtle. Have you ever been tricked into an intimate situation you did not desire? Has anyone ever touched you intimately against your will? Do you have a lot of trouble surrendering during lovemaking? Do you hate being touched? Do you have trouble setting boundaries with others? Do you find great difficulty in trusting others, especially members of the opposite sex? Do you continually find yourself stuck in relationships? Do you have a chronic illness, particularly a gynecological problem? Do you often feel outside yourself when you have sex? If these questions trigger even an inkling of response, contact a support organization and get help.

Sometimes, memories of abuse are triggered by stressful situations or life-changing events such as divorce, loss of home or income, natural disaster, death of a loved one, serious physical injury to oneself or a loved one, or physical violence of any kind. In short, anything that causes us to feel pushed to our limits and vulnerable is apt to release the subconscious and bring unpleasant memories to the surface.

This woman's story serves to illustrate:

> We were making love and were hot into it. My husband pushed me over on my side to enter me from behind, which I really didn't want, and suddenly, something just went off inside me and I panicked. Not in my head but in my heart, my gut, I felt this constriction, this fear. I knew it had nothing to do with him, but I couldn't deny the feeling. Actually, I had noticed this before in other situations with men when I felt they were manipulating me. I noticed the same fear and this feeling of terror, just below the surface. Part of me would freeze up and go limp, as if in survival mode.
>
> Finally, through hypnosis, I remembered some friend of my uncle's forcing me to let him play with my nipples, show him my backside and let him finger me, just a little on the outside. That's all that ever happened, but I responded in that same way back then—I froze, stood still, felt very much in danger but powerless to cry out. I felt totally humiliated, like I was no good, dirty, and it was all my fault.
>
> Once I got over this, I could see what was happening with my husband. Whenever he was forceful with me, even if it was really okay, I just froze up—I couldn't help it. And if I let him go ahead anyway, I had those same feelings of self-loathing. We had some stuff to work out, I can tell you!

In a moment, we will look further at how abuse affects sexuality. But first, here are some additional characteristics and modes of behavior common in women who have been abused.

- Describes self as never having been a child

- Extremely concerned with control

- Overly willing to expose genitals to others

- Unexplained pain with intercourse

- Extreme ideas about sexuality

- Hypersensitive to touch

- Repeatedly exploited by others in relationship

- Deeply estranged from family

- General feeling of being "under it"

- Detaches from self and others

- Nothing ever wrong with life, always neutral

- Childlike behavior, dress, or appearance

- Unkempt personal appearance

- Chaotic surroundings and habits

- Overly controlled surroundings or habits

- No personal boundaries

- No trust

- Anger inappropriate or out of proportion to the situation

○ Inability to appreciate others

○ Blind adoration of others

○ Fanatic religious or philosophical beliefs

○ Jumps into situations and to conclusions

○ Difficulty with decision making[1]

From this list, it is easy to extrapolate sexual response patterns of abusees, which range from total frigidity to compulsive sexual activity and display. The latter may be somewhat surprising, but it is as if the victim were saying, "See, I'm so sexual and out there with it that no one can take control of me—I'm in charge." This attitude generally precludes the surrender that leads to orgasm, and it almost certainly precludes intimacy. It bespeaks the stereotypical male approach to sex, that of using sex primarily for self-gratification and without the context of relationship. Women who have been abused may thus unconsciously reject their feminine vulnerability to be more on a par with their oppressor. Clarrise related, "In retrospect, it's like I bought into the beliefs of the man who abused me. My cunt was just a cunt, and I used it that way, keeping myself separate from it, using it as much as I could to prove the point that it was not me, I didn't have to be connected."

Psychological effects of abuse that increase vulnerability to disease, accidents, and other calamities are more difficult to track. Many characteristics of abusees are in fact contradictory, though decidedly extreme. Bipolar personality disorder often correlates to a history of sexual abuse.

Besides physical or sexual abuse, there are numerous other ways in which women are abused. Have you ever felt violated during a gynecological exam, by procedures or tools used forcibly to examine you when you clearly were not ready? Or, if you have given birth, did you feel in any way abused by procedures or technology used without your full consent and understanding? These types of abuse are less obvious because they are part of the cultural milieu, but the effects are the same: self-esteem and self-worth are diminished, personal boundaries are lost or disrupted, and sexual response and satisfaction are reduced.

In my many years of practicing women's health care, I have had ample experience with women suffering from what is commonly known as vaginismus: the uncontrollable contraction of vaginal muscles whenever penetration is attempted. This is especially sad to see in very young women, particularly if caused by an unnecessarily rough initial gynecological exam. These women may find it almost impossible to have intercourse, let alone regular checkups. Of course, vaginismus is also a classic sign of sexual abuse.

When working with a woman who has this problem, I go out of my way to put her in control. I suggest the use of a small speculum, and I teach her how to insert it herself. Sometimes this is not possible, and we need to stop, take a moment, then start again by having her put a finger inside to feel how her muscles contract so that she can work directly on relaxing them. This alone will not cure her condition; the same involuntary response will probably occur the next time she tries to have intercourse. But at least she may now have the confidence to continue to seek help, work on herself, and communicate her needs and fears to her partner.

If she cannot come to terms with her situation, she may find that the only way she can have sex is by disassociation. This is tragic because the pattern perpetuates itself, and the woman remains a victim.

Classic therapeutic techniques for vaginismus include behavioral approaches. The woman is asked to relax thoroughly and then imagine, step-by-step, the stages of intercourse while trying to stay open as much as possible. Sometimes plastic dilators are used by the woman herself to simulate penetration by another in conjunction with visualization.[2] The trouble with this approach is that it may not allow the necessary release of emotion, particularly of anger. Besides, penetration is not the be-all and end-all of sexual pleasure for women that it is for men. Penetration affords very little stimulation to the clitoris; thus women do not necessarily need penetration to find sexual fulfillment.

The best approach for a woman struggling with vaginismus is to talk with her partner and forge an exploration agreement. That is, the two of them agree to let her take the lead in showing her partner all the finer points of what is arousing to her, her particulars of pleasure. She can begin by showing him or her what she does when she masturbates, exactly where and how she likes to be touched. Then she can guide her partner to try the same—only that, and no more.

Kitzinger, who describes this technique in detail, recommends that from this point in the exchange, penetration occur only with the woman's own finger. Both the woman and her partner should agree in advance that she will be free to stop the process at any time. She must always be in control and in charge of the pace, doing as much as or as little as seems right to her each time. Some women find they actually prefer sex without penetration, and the couple then needs to work out some mutually acceptable arrangement.

In a similar vein are the traumas attendant on unplanned or undesired episiotomy when giving birth. As discussed in Chapter 5, there are practical considerations in healing the vaginal area when there has been injury or trauma, and most women who have had repair have a certain amount of hesitation the first time they have sex again. But some feel more than hesitation. The psychological trauma of episiotomy may link to a sense of violation—some women speak of feeling mutilated, changed, no longer themselves. The net result is similar to that of sexual abuse: the sufferer feels shame, guilt, and inadequacy after having been violated, as if it were all her fault.

Whatever abuse a woman has experienced, working through it demands that she relive the event while being witnessed by a third party so that her reactions can be vented, explored, and recast. Northrup concurs: "Lower chakra [sexual] wounds don't heal until they're witnessed."[3] Unfortunately, many victims of abuse never have the opportunity to be heard, and they remain full of repressed anger. Without validation for their fury and humiliation, they turn these feelings on themselves, in self-abnegation.

The healing process must also incorporate factual information about abuse, enough to help a woman see her trauma in the larger social context—she must realize that she is not the only one to whom this kind of violation has occurred! Ultimately, she needs support in releasing the power her wounds have held over her life. This seldom takes place overnight.

Emotional Abuse

Whatever happens to a woman's body also happens to her spirit. Thus, emotional abuse is an undeniable component of physical abuse. When a woman is raped, she suffers much more than physical injury. Feelings of terror and utter powerlessness combined with the threats or insults of her attacker have as far-reaching effects as does the degradation of her body. Girls who are victims of incest likewise feel the psychological manipulations of a trusted relative to be just as devastating as the physical violation.

But emotional abuse may also stand alone, often manifesting in negative patterns of relationship that tend to repeat themselves. And since both sexes are susceptible to the emotional manipulations of others, we must look beyond misogyny for causes.

We can trace some of our susceptibility to emotional abuse back to early childhood experience, particularly as regards attachment to our parents. According to Avodah Offit, M.D., author of *The Sexual Self*, sexual behavior is very much influenced by the degree to which we have bonded to another in infancy, which in turn affects how well we tolerate the anxiety of separation. If we are kept close and secure when young, we become more comfortable with ourselves as we mature and are better able to handle being alone. If, as stated by William James, "The greatest terror of infancy is solitude," perhaps we must reassess our ways of fostering independence in our young. Putting our children on their own at an early age has not worked, for us or them. It has been a survival strategy, an adaptation in a culture moving too fast for intimate relationship. But our need to attach to others and to depend on them is perfectly normal. The more healthy and sound our early attachments, the less susceptible we are to unhealthy, compulsive/abusive relationships.

A great turning point and reckoning in this regard occurs when we first fall in love. Separation anxiety becomes intense as we realize that in bonding and attaching so deeply to another, our bonds to our parents will be forever changed. Our need to be close, to be protected and to protect, are suddenly transferred to someone new.

Ideally, separation anxiety and the concomitant desire for closeness motivate us to endure the challenging stages of intimate relationship. It might well be said that a strong bond in infancy with our mother or other loving adult is our only real basis for meeting life's onslaughts with courage and equanimity. If this initial attachment is hindered, things predictably go awry; our subsequent attachments are apt to be inhibited or fragmented. The less we are able to connect with and trust others, the greater our anxiety and dependence. It is thus that we become ready targets for emotional abuse.

Even if our original attachments are sound, we are so vulnerable when first in love that reimprinting may occur. As mentioned in Chapter 2, psychologist Alfred Ellis suggests that we can often trace unsatisfying and dysfunctional patterns in relationship to our first sexual interaction. Here are some questions that might help you evaluate your own experience. Did your first love share his/her heart with you, or just his/her body? Was he/she patient and kind, or uncaring and inconsiderate? Was he/she honest and forthright with you, or deceiving and untrue? Did the relationship end amicably or with unresolved anger, pain, and humiliation? Did you feel in any way abused by him/her?

Emotional abuse is thus defined as any behavior designed to control or subjugate another through emotionally based techniques of intimidation, ridicule, invalidation, manipulation, or verbal assault. Sometimes it's easier to recognize the effects of emotional abuse than the contributing behavior. If you suffer from low self-esteem, mistrust of your perceptions, inability to appreciate your accomplishments, lack of motivation, chronic depression, or difficulty in taking charge of your life, you are probably a victim.

Keep in mind that emotional abuse can take many forms. I've worked with women, otherwise confident and secure, who have been utterly devastated by a partner's assessment that their vagina is either too loose, too tight, too long, or too short, that their sexual intensity is not up to par, or that their nipples are not pink enough, large enough, hard enough, and so on. I am both frustrated and saddened by the frequency with which women question the adequacy of their bodies, the appearance of breasts and genitals that are perfectly normal. It is important to remember that sexual domination victimizes us as surely as more direct forms of abuse.

It is also crucial that we not minimize the effects of coercion—another common strategy of emotional abusers. Whenever an intimate partner makes us feel inadequate as a means to control, or tries to place the locus of responsibility on us for his or her happiness, we are looking at emotional abuse.

Five Profiles of Abusees

In *The Emotionally Abused Woman,* Beverly Engel presents five distinct profiles of chronic abusees, each of which finds a complement in a particular type of abuser. Abusers can be anyone in a role of authority: parents, teachers, bosses, mentors, or religious leaders. They may also be peer counterparts such as siblings, co-workers, friends, or lovers.[4]

Note that these abuser/abusee configurations are not sequential and have no rank of superiority or inferiority. But all too often, women move from one configuration to another. The main thing these abusee roles have in common is that they align with feelings of powerlessness and inadequacy. Women are most apt to step into one of these roles just as they begin to care deeply for someone, for it is precisely at this point that their deep conditioning is triggered.

Here, then, are five profiles of abusees. There are similarities among the first four, but subtle differences arise in the sort of partner each type of woman tends to select.

Selfless and Silent
The selfless and silent woman has usually been dominated, controlled, or neglected in her young years to such an extreme degree that she has little or no sense of self. She may take on the personality of others,

particularly when in love—anything to be accepted. On the other hand, intimacy is both frightening and threatening to her.

When it comes to sex, she moves in and out of relationships with great frequency. Sex tends either to be deeply inhibited or explosive, releasing deep and overwhelming emotions that cannot be integrated. Women stuck in this role are in a turmoil when in love, empty when not. As one of my clients confided to me:

> I don't really know how to be close to a man, but I sure do try. Usually I try to be like him, doing what he likes to do, even in bed, no matter what. Sometimes I feel hurt, used, and very sad, and then I get so pissed off and furious I have to leave. I hate that, though, because when I'm by myself I feel so empty. That scares me so much I start looking for someone else right away.

Under these circumstances, intimacy is forever elusive. As Avodah Offit observes, "In bed, dependence more often leads to erotic extinction than to an eternal flame of passion."[5] A woman of silent/selfless temperament is usually attracted to her opposite—a highly self-involved type with little or no ability to care for another. The longer she stays with a partner like this, the more she is apt to be drawn into his or her narcissistic, grandiose schemes. If and when she decides to leave, she will have to cope with the loss of all she has invested, plus a further diminished sense of self.

Women thus afflicted need professional help through hypnosis, long-term therapy, or other deep work to trace patterns of self-abuse back to their original source.

Servile and Compulsive

Women in the servile and compulsive role are also excessively dependent, centered on the expectations of others. Almost every woman today has some "pleaser" in her, so deeply ingrained is the cultural expectation that we put others' needs before our own. However, the servile/compulsive woman takes this to an extreme, and she will tolerate and suffer the demeaning and abusive behavior of others to an extent that is utterly damaging to all concerned. Just as she blames herself for the misdeeds of her intimates, she likewise impedes them from taking responsibility for their own actions. If she happens on a moment of clarity and notices how others take advantage of her, she usually begins apologizing for her own behavior, repressing herself and remaining dependent.

Why does a woman behave thus? Typically, her parents demanded perfection and consistently ignored her personal boundaries and limits. Perhaps she was berated simply for being female. Whatever the cause, she is unlikely to find happiness in bed. She is generally far too busy evaluating her performance, trying to assess it by her partner's standards. "Was it good enough?" she queries, "Was I okay, are you sure it was really all right?" Unlike the silent/selfless type, she rarely knows the benefits of explosive release. She is continually in a quandary with regard to her adequacy: preoccupied, distracted from herself, intent on measuring up. She may conversely avoid sex altogether and focus her obsessive anxiety on her career, her children's accomplishments, the cleanliness of her house, and so on. In short, she is mortally afraid of losing control, of letting the monster of her own frustrated needs and desires out of the bag.

Typically, she does not reach orgasm with intercourse. There are many reasons a woman might not have an orgasm, but in this case, the servile/compulsive woman cannot connect with herself enough to let go. For her, the *petite morte* of orgasm is downright terrifying. As Karen related:

> I try to give my lover everything she wants in bed—I give
> and give until honestly, I feel weak and sick inside. Nothing

I do seems to really excite her, and when she finally comes, I start worrying about what she's thinking and whether or not I've really pleased her. I know I shouldn't say this, but I'd rather put my energy into the house or my work, where I know I can do some good.

Ironically, this woman is often paired with a controlling type, one who continually reinforces her need to please by being hypercritical.

The servile/compulsive woman needs to learn that life is not about meeting some outside standard of perfection; it's about loving and developing the Self. She must practice putting herself first, letting go, and having fun (it won't come naturally). This often involves attaching some name or face from the past to the censoring voice of her inner critic. Her primary key to happiness is reconnecting with her wild, original self, then getting back on her own track in life. Sexually, she will need a new foundation based on her own needs and desires. She may need professional help with this.

Guilt-Ridden and Reactive

The guilt-ridden and reactive role is otherwise known as that of the sinner. The woman playing it is more physically expressive than the other types we've discussed, but her passions bring nothing but guilt and shame. She is so burdened with self-loathing that she barely relates to her partner; sex holds no intimacy for her. Women in this pattern are often victims of physical and/or severe emotional abuse, taught to believe their inherent naughtiness, seductiveness, or worthlessness are just cause for their violation. As adults, they are in reaction to these imprints. Engel puts it most succinctly: "Sinners believe that bad things only happen to bad people."[6]

Guilt-ridden/reactive women typically choose partners who reinforce their guilt by blaming them for everything under the sun, which only perpetuates their feelings of unworthiness. Blamers may themselves be passionate and reactive, unrealistic and unstable—they may even be closet sinners. But whoever plays the role of blamer is always right, the sinner, always wrong.

As Sharon revealed, "My boyfriend says terrible things to me sometimes, and I know I should forgive him but I just can't. Then I see even more how he's right—I really am a terrible person. I don't do the shopping on time because I want to read instead, or I forget to pay bills because I'm out with my friends." What about her sex life? "I really like sex, but I get pretty scared and nervous about it sometimes. If I mess up, I cry and have to stop, I feel so awful inside, and he tells me it's all my fault. He's right, of course, but that just makes it worse. Sometimes I go out with other guys and it's better, but I'm scared that my boyfriend will find out. The truth is, I like sex, but I hate what it does to me."

The guilt-ridden/reactive woman absorbs her partner's ills and delusions without discrimination. Their relationship is so volatile and out of balance that she rightly equates love with pain. She must learn how to distinguish positive, life-affirming passions from negative, destructive ones. She must start listening to her own voice, seeing her worth apart from the opinions of others. She must rid herself of shadows, those of blamers past and present. Frequently, there is history of alcoholism or drug abuse in the family, and she, her partner, or both are dependent. Professional help is once again in order.

Passive and Victimized

Women in a passive role are targets for victimization and tragedy. Sexually, they are easily manipulated and apt to be used, perpetually finding themselves in the wrong place at the wrong time with the wrong person. The victim's life is ridden with anxiety; she is extremely susceptible to the maneuvers of others. Frequently, she partners with those who seek to disempower her by systematically invalidating her actions and perceptions. The more she is invalidated, the greater her passivity and dependency.

Since her intimate partners have full sway, she is often the victim of their verbal or physical abuse. The victim tells herself she deserves it because she's inept or just crazy. Frequently, she witnessed a similar pattern at home.

This woman's partner is often a bit of a sociopath, living for sexual conquest without any hint of regard for his partner. Typically, the sociopath is admired by all—except for those who have seen through him. Deviously and methodically, he manipulates his partner into submission. He won't respond to her advances but nevertheless insists that she respond to his. He bestows his affection on her only when she is extremely busy, and then accuses her of being cold and unresponsive. He may even make her question her sanity by pretending never to have said or done things he said or did quite deliberately. He is a master at making others feel uncomfortable while seeming to do nothing at all.[7] (Of course, women can also play the sexual sociopath role in lesbian partnerships.)

With a sociopath, sex will go only one way: their own. They are completely in charge, calling all the shots. The victim will feel ignorant and inadequate, convinced there is something seriously wrong with her sexual abilities. As Julie says:

> The only time sex was any good for me was when we were making up—it gave me a chance to express my love to Gene, to reassure myself that he still loved me. The rest of the time I felt too insecure to make any moves in bed, and I don't think Gene wanted me to anyway—I had so many problems. Sometimes, though, I let him force me into it. I suffered through, hoping I could improve myself in his eyes.

Passive victim types may be helped with support groups. Counseling is crucial, and social support, including legal assistance, is essential if physical violence has occurred.

Hysterical and Overdrawn

The hysterical and overdrawn woman is the last type we will consider. The word *hysterical* derives from the Latin word for *uterus*, and common use of the term harks back to a time when irrational or highly excitable women were believed to be under the influence of uterine "ethers" moving about their body. The somewhat less derogatory term *histrionic* is now more commonly used. I rather like the term *hysterical* because it implies a woman under the influence of feminine energies and forces, albeit to an extreme.

Women thus oriented thrive on intensity, high drama, and chaos. From an early age they were either strictly controlled and inhibited or wracked with constant crisis and disruption. Either way, these women feel most alive and comfortable in the midst of (or while making) a scene. They consistently seek situations that engender strong emotions like anger or jealousy—anything to stir things up a bit. They frequently choose unstable partners in unstable circumstances. There is a strong tendency to upset the balance continually or to become involved in confrontations that are irreconcilable.

When it comes to love and sex, a woman of this kind will generally choose unwisely, perhaps a severely antisocial partner or a near psychopath. She may be attracted to a substance abuser, compulsive gambler, sex addict, or someone in trouble with the law. She may go for the "hard cases," individuals so disturbed that they are nearly impossible to reach. She may also choose someone unavailable (married, for example) or clearly not interested. She is not apt to select a healthy, somewhat normal person with a decent likelihood of loving her and treating her respectfully.

The hysterical and overdrawn woman uses drama as a smoke screen to avoid looking at her problems. Her partner is doing the same; it is the main thing they have in common. Tension is her drug, and she uses it to keep chaos at a level that feels familiar and comfortable. Setting ultimatums, staging rescues and arguments, she makes her partner's problems her own, creating so much stress in their relationship that abuse may come as a welcome release.

Sexually, it's a roller coaster. This woman's counterpart usually has a highly volatile personality, which may be further intensified by drugs, alcohol, intrigue, or criminal activity. Sex can be unbelievably hot and explosive, at the same time riddled with cruelty and manipulation. The most noticeably absent quality in both partners is genuine vulnerability.

Here's a typical report:

> The best thing about our relationship was the sex. I loved to entice Jack into sex when he wasn't really in the mood. Sometimes I'd have to make a scene, accuse and argue with him just to get him angry and really hot for me. Then he'd take me to the limit, and I'd scream and holler my way to oblivion. Other times he was cold, cruel, and calculating. If I let him make love to me like that, he would trick me out— you know, make it hard for me to come, or make me come when I wasn't ready. I'd be so angry, I'd pull way back. Then he would apologize, and we'd have blowout sex again.

Note the contradictions here: on the one hand, sex was "the best thing," on the other hand, it was degrading. Clearly, this woman must learn to find stability and security within herself. She must learn to use her lust for excitement in constructive ways, or she is destined for serious burnout. To do this, she needs a counselor's help. Even if not drug or alcohol dependent herself, she may benefit from contact with an abusers' or a family of alcoholics' group, exploring the characteristics of relationship under the shadow of dependency.

* * *

If we are honest with ourselves, we will all admit that we have played at least one of these roles to some extent in our lives. Whether we have experienced emotional or physical abuse, or both, the bottom line is the same: we must acknowledge and effectively address it. Remember what was said earlier, too, about the need to be witnessed.

However, we must also give ourselves permission to do as much or as little work on these issues as feels right at any given time. Any woman who has been forced or compelled into intimate contact against her best interests must feel free to follow her instincts in this regard. Healing work is rhythmic: two steps forward, one step back, rather like birthing a baby. If we push it, we may sink back into feelings of powerlessness and inertia.

Sexual Addiction

Let us not confuse sexual addiction with a healthy appetite for intimacy! Some women want and have sex several times a day, especially in the early stages of relationship.

When we fall in love, most of us long for our partners so much that we can hardly endure physical separation. This is not an addiction, but bonding, healthy attachment behavior.

It bears mentioning, though, that there is new evidence that women may not be as monogamous by nature as previously thought.

Biologically, the fact that male sperm are not merely egg-seeking but have block and attack mechanisms against alien sperm suggests an adaptation made to females with more than one partner.[8]

And how, before the advent of contraception, could women be so free without being found out? The answer is that frequent childbearing and breast-feeding rendered women anovulatory for long enough periods that they could easily be with a number of partners without consequence of pregnancy. This was particularly true of hunter-gatherer women, reportedly so active that they rarely ovulated.[9]

There are also numerous pre-Christian traditions that honored women who were sexually wise. These women were the sexual initiators of men, in the tradition of the vestal virgins of ancient Greece, or the sacred *dakinis* of the East. Studies of our prehistory also reveal numerous figures of women either displaying their genitals or opening them to view, like Kali of India or Sheila-na-gig of Celtic traditions.[10] Women who find that they impart to others profound wisdom though sexual contact, especially if the experience feels sacred and happens to them repeatedly, will undoubtedly have an unconventional sexual history involving many partners.

But when sex is a drug used to avoid difficulties in life, or to find validation that should come from inside, we have a problem. It's a fine line: we all use sex occasionally for reassurance or to meet our most basic needs for intimate contact. But when sexual activity undermines our work or professional relationships, or when it is hurtful to others, sexuality is no longer in its proper life-affirming place.

Consider this case history of a woman caught in compulsive sexual behavior. Tina reported a tempestuous and stressful phase in a career she wanted to escape; she was overworked and completely exhausted. She met up with an old friend, now married, and despite her better judgment, started sleeping with him. In her words:

> It's not like we were in love. I felt comfortable with him, and it was a fantastic release. But the more we did it, the less I felt. I don't know how to describe it; it was like I was numb, emotionally dead inside. Still, he took good care of me, got me nice things, all that. . . .
>
> Then, of all things, I got pregnant! I'd only been pregnant once before and this was a complete accident, total carelessness. It shocked me into seeing what I was doing . . . I wasn't taking care of myself at all, I was just using sex to get by. So I had an abortion and ended the relationship.

Here, an otherwise assertive woman became a passive victim in relationship. Work-related stress, uncertainty about her future, and inability to deal with impending changes in her life led to self-destructive behavior.

Another example from Janelle, married with a child:

> My husband was the classic executive, straight-arrow, in his head and anxious all the time. After our son was born, sex just stopped. I felt like I had dried up inside, that I was losing my beauty and my charm. I started an affair with a man in the neighborhood—he was unemployed and his wife worked—I even knew her slightly. He had problems, and I tried to help. It was so wonderful to be needed, to be admired, to have that hot kind of sex that is just so good! But after a while I started seeing him for what he was—a loser, pure and simple, and somebody else's husband. Quite suddenly I saw that I'd been using him to avoid the disappointment I felt in my own marriage, and my anxiety about finding a life of my own. It was a rude awakening to have to look at things I'd been putting off for a long time.

Examples like this are common enough. Then again, sexual addiction may link to an insatiable sexual appetite, a condition we call nymphomania. Sexologists generally concur that nymphomania results from a lack of healthy attachment and separation experiences. Nymphomaniacs can't bear to be alone; they desperately crave the comforts of human contact, presumably to compensate for some deprivation experienced when they were young.

Most of us have known or heard of women who consistently bed new partners, who are always "on the make." These women typically have such high anxiety levels that intercourse, no matter how frequent, doesn't make a dent in their insecurity. Although some are multiorgasmic and may climax twenty or more times in one experience, others report orgasms as unfulfilling and monotonous. The vast majority is rarely orgasmic. The out-of-control aspect of the nymphomaniac's behavior makes it nearly impossible for her to let go. In short, nymphomaniacs are in general profoundly immature, deeply injured, and repressed.

For women with a history of sexual addiction, or of sexual or emotional abuse, an admittedly unconventional option for healing is to forego sex altogether until the ground is set for healthier patterns of intimacy. In the next chapter, we will look at celibacy as an increasingly common choice for women trying to rid themselves of destructive sexual behaviors.

Celibacy

A Time for
Loving Yourself

Women who decide to abstain from sex, for whatever reason, have been looked upon by our society as something of an anomaly. To be sexually active is so deeply ingrained in our recipe for happiness that a woman without a partner is presumed to be longing and deprived. As we will see in the forthcoming pages, nothing could be further from the truth, at least when abstinence is a choice.

In fact, a growing number of women choose to take a break from sexual activity when personal issues or problems intervene. This coincides with great gains over the last century in women's social and economic autonomy. Cultural constraints that once put the reins of a woman's sexual activity in the hands of her male provider no longer hold sway. Women may be still be viewed as sex objects, but increasingly are shown by the media to have sexual identities of their own. It is no longer unacceptable that women choose, particularly under circumstances of stress or emotional strain, to set sex aside in order to conserve their vital energies.

To illustrate, here is my own story. It was about 1982, and my ex-husband and I were going through a particularly difficult time in our relationship; we were not yet married (a bone of contention between us) and were working out negative consequences of an affair he'd had at the beginning of our relationship. That these issues had disrupted our sex life seemed quite natural to me, although I won't deny I was concerned. Our therapist, a supposed expert in sexual dysfunction, somehow thought it necessary to show us a video of a couple engaged in foreplay, with step-by-step instructions. This experience both mortified and infuriated me, and I told her outright, "I don't need this, I don't think we have any problems with technique. My problem is with my feelings, my pain and vulnerability, the trust issue. If we work on these, maybe I'll want to have sex again."

This is not to minimize sex therapy for those with unusual aversions or compulsions, but for the vast majority of women, sexual dysfunction is emotionally based, nothing more. We don't need another survey to tell us that a woman cannot be loving, open, and orgasmic if she feels her partner is treating (or has treated) her poorly or unfairly, let alone if she feels she can't be heard.

What is it like to take a sexual time-out? Depends on the situation, but most women report initial loneliness and/or relief, followed by renewed self-confidence and clarity. Brenda, a single woman in her thirties, tells how a series of relationships frightened her into abstinence that then became voluntary for a period of seven months:

> I had an outrageous affair with a fellow who turned out to be royalty, a Scottish lord in fact. It was a whirlwind romance, and in a matter of weeks he proposed marriage. On the one hand, I knew I'd be taken care of for life, and all my friends were telling me to go for it. But this is a pattern that keeps repeating in my life—guys go crazy for me, and the situation becomes overwhelming. Maybe I have something to do with it—after all, I let it happen, to a point. Then I feel this pressure of being swept away, and I just pull back or quit. I do notice that it happens more when I'm unsettled or stressed at work.
>
> So, I said no to this guy with much relief; then the same thing happened with a man who turned out to be married—there were signs and signals that I never followed up until it was way too late. After this I pulled back completely from men and sex.
>
> Being celibate all this time has given me some important things. One is protection—I can feel vulnerable with myself and not be at risk. Another is a very clear picture of what I

want in relationship—marriage to the right man. Eventually, because now I'm content to wait.

Other comments from women in similar circumstances: "I'm pleased and proud to be nurturing me," "I see the seeds of myself beginning to grow," "I have inner conviction now—I'm my own person." Voluntary abstinence may thus be a rite of passage for women today, particularly in response to tremendously eased sexual mores.

Yet another factor in women's choice of celibacy is their desire to reconnect with their bodies and feel their own rhythms. In other cultures, women had (or have) regular opportunity for a physical time-out via isolation during menstruation. Whatever other effects this isolation may have incurred, it definitely got women away from their male partners for a few days so they could disentangle themselves from routine obligations and reflect on personal issues. Perhaps we all need such a respite, a chance to keep body and soul to ourselves periodically without guilt or anxiety. Without this, we may get stuck in patterns of self-denial and subservience.

As Lynda explains:

> I grew up in a household where Mom's main task was taking care of everyone else's business. I loved her for it, hated her for it, learned to depend on her and not myself. Even though we fought bitterly when I was in my teens, I found myself continually dependent and wanting to please her before myself. Three marriages and three children later, I still don't know all that much about me. My sexuality has been confined, I think, to what's been expected.
>
> I've been abstinent for three months now, and it's been a good way for me to sort things out and get to the heart of who I am. To tell you the truth, I feel like a kid again,

discovering broken threads from the past and reweaving them. Right now, I don't want anyone else but me.

This again points to a need of women throughout time, that of self-containment, a "room of one's own." In *Women and Madness*, Phyllis Chesler reveals how diffusing the self for the ease and pleasure can cause a complete disintegration of personality.[1] When a woman is able to rally from this extreme it is usually with passion and fury, a passion that requires no other partner than herself.

Other times, sexual excess leads to celibacy. This, too, is a classic theme, and women are not exempt. Here is what Alena has to say:

> I was fairly repressed when I was young, living in a house that was immaculately clean and bound by strict rules of behavior. There was love, but there was also fear; I guess my mom was afraid of herself, and of us kids too, what we might do. I took the road less traveled (at least in my family) and dropped out of school. I met wild and wonderful people, and found I could make good money selling sexual favors . . . not prostitution exactly, but I'd give intimate massages, blow jobs, that kind of thing. I was choosy, though, and never a slave to anyone. For a while I felt free, for the first time in my life. Then good friends turned bad, a few died of drug overdoses, and I turned to religion. I needed to purify myself, and I didn't have sex with anyone for three years.

As we enter our third decade of coping with HIV and AIDS, plus hepatitis B and C, stories like this become increasingly rare. Sexual addiction and overindulgence nonetheless remain major pathways to celibacy for a number of women.

More commonly, women choose celibacy because they feel prostituted in seemingly conventional relationships. Often this comes from repressing the pain of unmet needs, of feeling ignored or belittled. As the relationship deteriorates, sex usually becomes sporadic: a few encounters once in a while, then weeks with no contact. Interestingly, research has shown that sporadic sexual activity is more likely to cause menstrual irregularity and subfertility than is celibacy. Masturbation (even to orgasm) does not seem to compensate. Either regular sex, or none at all, tends to maintain normal hormonal levels and rhythms.[2]

Unless a couple has an agreement that their relationship is open, nothing disrupts sexual closeness like infidelity. Trust is so basic to a healthy relationship that if it is violated, intimacy may be impossible to regain without separation and time to heal. Again, a classic account, from Harriet:

> My husband was unfaithful from day one, but it took me years to acknowledge this. Once I did, I went crazy with jealousy and fear. I started having anxiety attacks; I just couldn't control myself. I'd be at the bank or in some store, and suddenly I'd feel dizzy, breathless, light-headed—my heart would be racing and I'd have to sit down.
>
> I ended my marriage, but then, the same thing happened with the next guy. I finally realized that sex had become so fearsome and painful for me that I'd probably keep losing again and again, unless I broke the cycle on my own. So I quit looking for the right man, for perfect romance, and got down to being by myself. Some days I felt so alone that panic nearly got me again, but eventually I could catch these feelings and get rid of them right away. I discovered things that nourished me and made me feel complete, instead of trying to fit other people's notions of what I should be.

Pain and heartbreak aside, it is time for women to recognize that the sexes definitely differ in erotic temperament. According to research presented by Anne Moir and David Jessel in *Brain Sex*, there is convincing evidence that men are by nature polygamous and tend to focus on sex for its own sake.[3] This does not preclude romance or even monogamous commitment, but a woman should know what she is up against. In any case, happiness comes not from seeking some idealized version of masculinity, but in accepting men as they are. Relationships involve conflict because male and female desires appear to be at odds, but they may also be viewed as complementary. Each has gender-based needs that are fairly consistent; John Gray has illuminated this quite well. For example, women need to feel cared for and loved in order to be able to trust their partners. Men need to feel trusted in order to care; a man without a woman's trust loses his momentum and his vitality. Men will invariably fail to care for us as we would like, and we will likewise lose trust in them, but that doesn't change the basic needs of each. The more realistic we are about our differences, and the more we accept our own traits and tendencies, the better we will be at weathering the ups and downs in relationships, the inevitable challenges and disappointments.

When a woman chooses sexual abstinence, she has an opportunity to own both her masculine and feminine aspects and bring them to terms with each other. For example, she can look at how much love and nourishment she gives herself, and, if minimal, the resulting lack of trust and vulnerability she is able to offer others. This will not change her basic needs in a relationship: no matter how well she has learned to care for herself, she will still be susceptible to being hurt by an uncaring partner. But she may be better equipped to deal with disappointments and estrangement when they occur, and go on caring for herself regardless.

How constructive a period of abstinence is for a woman largely depends on how deliberate it is. When abstinence is by choice, negative side effects like depression may not occur. If depression does enter the picture, watch for signs that it is worsening, such as lack of motivation, flat moods, and disinterest in personal hygiene. Counseling can help, as can time spent regularly with other women in a group process or circle.

One reason women do not find much cultural support for celibacy is that men find sex a prerequisite for emotional release, a precursor to love. Women, on the other hand, are more readily able to love themselves and others without sexual demonstration. When women choose celibacy, they threaten male needs and male control; we see this reflected in our language by terminology that is far from flattering, such as *old maid, spinster,* and *prude.*

Thus some women worry about remaining physically attractive without the benefits of sexual contact. But celibacy does not preclude pleasuring yourself, and masturbation offers numerous benefits, not the least of which is stress relief. It also stimulates pelvic circulation, which helps keep the pelvic organs in good health. Then again, there are innumerable ways to find physical and emotional release unrelated to sex. Some women just don't want sex, whatever the reason, and that's all there is to it.

What, if any, are the physical effects of long-term abstinence? Some women report symptoms of pelvic tension such as chronic backache, increased PMS, or menstrual difficulties, but just as many report cessation of these problems, particularly when abstinent after ending a miserable relationship. Occasionally, women report losing touch with the monthly cycle, becoming less aware of fertile and premenstrual signals. If fertility awareness was used as a contraceptive method, this is certainly understandable. Perhaps women who think they have lost touch are busy subconsciously revising emotional and spiritual aspects of cycling to suit their newfound autonomy.

Many women notice increased awareness of diet and health when on their own. Without the distraction of caring for another, they are better able to see the results of their own nutrition and lifestyle habits, and to experiment with what makes them feel best. Particularly if a woman has been living with someone and cooking and eating more to suit his or her wishes than her own, she may find this aspect of being alone most illuminating and beneficial.

Women often report that the less sex they have, the less they think about it. At times, the longing for contact is strong, but usually it is more a desire for intimacy than for sex itself (unless a woman is peak-fertile or premenstrual). Celibacy is really less about sex than it is about solitude, learning to deal with one's own body, psyche, and soul.

Other reasons why a woman might choose to avoid sex temporarily have little to do with relationship. A friend recently shared plans for a yearlong trip around the world, along with her decision to forego sexual involvement until after she left—no dates, no serious flirting, just packing and settling affairs. Similar motivations might be plans to relocate, change careers, or focus on a creative project. When taken as a spiritual discipline, celibacy has long been reputed to enhance energy and concentration.

What if a woman elects to take this option in spite of the fact that she is married or in relationship? We read and hear much about differences in sexual desire between partners, and, at last, the periodic desire for abstinence is coming out of the closest. Surveys on sexual frequency in committed relationships can be intimidating and therefore discouraging of this, but remember, these surveys deal in averages only; they do not address the quality of sexual interactions, nor do they exclude the flurry of activity typical in the early stages of relationship, when major challenges to intimacy have yet to be faced. I can think of no long-term study that truly reflects phases of closeness and separation in enduring relationships.

How does a couple get by when one wants sex and the other does not? Ideally, they discuss the matter, make some agreements, and set some limits. If this does not work, they need outside help. Marriages in distress are frequently challenged to redefine sex from an obligatory or perfunctory activity to one based on free will. Periodic abstinence may be crucial to sorting out individual needs and rhythms. And if either partner has been unfaithful or emotionally or physically abusive to the other, so much more the case. After all, what possible tenderness, joy, or security could come from sexual contact under such tenuous circumstances?

Personal traumas are also likely to interfere with a couple's sex life—particularly the loss of a loved one. The death of a child, a parent or other relative, or a dear friend may cause either a desperate need for contact or complete disinterest. If only one partner is affected, the other may provide stable ground. But if both are devastated, the emotional intensity of sex may be just too much to handle. Rhythms of processing grief are often at odds, so that when one partner is raw and vulnerable, the other is shut down and unable to feel much of anything. Here is Amanda's story of what happened to her after the death of her son at eight weeks from crib death, or SIDS (Sudden Infant Death Syndrome):

> I don't think there is anything more horribly painful on earth than losing a child—at least, I hope there's not, because I don't think I could endure it. Jerry and I had many sad and upsetting experiences trying to make love after Jason's death, but this one time was so amazing I must share it with you. We were fucking and crying, really, fucking and crying, when we felt something descend on us, a deep break in the tension, a feeling of warmth and healing. It was so wonderful, I can't tell you . . . like we were in a perfect state of grace. Sex aside, orgasm aside, in that moment, time stood still and we were okay again. After this, we stopped doubting and blaming ourselves so much. The guilt began to lift, and we began to live day by day.

Reestablishing intimacy after any kind of intensely painful experience or shock is a difficult process; this couple was lucky to find
common ground. Time heals, but the road is rocky and uneven.
Realigning ourselves after deep trauma is hardly a simple matter; layer
upon layer must be permeated with new hope and resolve. Once we
encouraged survivors to express their grief profoundly and immediately, believing that if they did so, they would be over it; now we know
that mourning is in fact a cyclical process and may extend for years and
years, even a lifetime. The same is true, by the way, for anyone recov-
ering from experiences of physical, emotional, or sexual abuse. Tina
relates:

> Pat and I had known each other for about a year, while
> she was still living with her former partner. Then she and I
> became intimate, and she decided to leave Sue. She felt a
> lot of guilt about this decision, along with sadness and
> confusion regarding her patterns of passivity from childhood
> abuse. Just as she became free to be with me, she decided
> she couldn't be sexual for a while. That was okay; I under-
> stood.

Coping with the effects of debilitating illness, handicap, or muti-
lating surgery such as mastectomy or hysterectomy may also call for a
sexual time off.

Sometimes the desire for abstinence becomes permanent, as in
Joan's case:

> I'm sixty-nine now, and my husband died six years ago. A
> couple of years after his death, friends tried to set me up with
> men, and at first I was curious, interested. But each time it
> was so obviously wrong that all I felt was revulsion. I'd think
> to myself, "I have to get in bed with that?" I had such a

wonderful marriage, and now I have my children and grand-children. I've got used to being alone, and honestly, I like it.

At the other end of spectrum is the simple desire to wait for the right relationship. More and more women are choosing to remain virgins late into their teens or throughout their early twenties, no longer feeling so intense a pressure to prove their sexual abilities. This has much to do with living in the shadow of AIDS and other sexually transmitted diseases.

Thus, for the first time in modern history, women have the freedom to choose from a spectrum of sexual options. Now that sex by coercion is defined as abuse, and sex by obligation is becoming passé, we are further free to acknowledge ourselves as sexual beings even if celibate. The prime dictum of sex therapy—"Don't worry about pleasing your partner, start by pleasing yourself"—may soon be realized by women on a mass scale. Women will find that their sexual energy is vital to their own well-being, instrumental to their creativity, health, and happiness, whether shared with another or not. Indeed, it will seem increasingly natural and normal that a woman (or man) might have times in life when sexual interaction is either inappropriate, undesirable, or low on the list of priorities, and that there will also be times when we elect to channel our sexual energy into personal pursuits.

Personal Passages

*Discovering Your
Own Sexual
Journey*

How you make use of the material in this book depends on many things, not the least of which are any unresolved issues of abuse, grief, or loss. These so strongly affect your receptivity and sense of self that they almost certainly will overshadow natural changes at different stages of life.

And yet, as we live each day and notice the turning of the cycles in our lives, we also begin to observe certain things about ourselves, ways in which we remain troubled or inhibited—our toughest challenges. The more creatively and constructively we are able to work on these, the richer and more multidimensional our experience at the next stage of life will be.

This closing chapter is written workbook style, with specific questions intended to shed light on these psychosexual patterns. Rather than allow blank space for writing within the book, I encourage you to use separate paper. The questions are provocative and intimately revealing, and I doubt you would want someone browsing through your bookshelves to come across your responses.

But do write your answers down! Committing yourself in writing is altogether different from musing, even if aloud. As you write, you may notice certain words that keep cropping up, or phrases from the treasure box of your past that have deep and vivid meaning for you. Or you may find empty expressions that you might wish to rethink or change.

If you would like to evoke your personal sentiments more strongly, you might choose a colored pen that best represents your mood during a particular period and write with it. Or design a symbol—an open circle, a spiral, a caricature of your totem animal, whatever—that represents your feelings at that particular stage, and place it at the top of your page. Your symbol can certainly change during a given cycle; you may well find that it does. If you have a tarot deck, select a card at critical junctures that embodies your feelings and beliefs, and make a note of it. You may also change your name as you write, to a nickname or private "soul" name that no one knows but you.

The journey through the labyrinth of sexuality is not only personal, it is mythic. Don't be afraid to lend this dimension of value and significance to the intimate details of your life.

Sexual Awakening

See if you can get in touch with your history here, tracing back your sexual attitudes, inhibitions, and expectations. Go back to the beginning: How did you learn about sex? Were you given a chance to question as fully as you desired? How did those you questioned respond to you? Do you remember the first time you masturbated? What was your first orgasm like? How was your first experience of sexual experimentation with another? Your first experience of intercourse? How did you feel about each of these experiences?

How did you learn about menstruation? What was your menarche like—was it hidden from the rest of your family and friends, or acknowledged in some positive way?

You may wish to recast these events in a more positive framework. Even if you had no celebration at your menarche, it is never too late. What would you like this celebration to include? I know a woman who recently crafted and held a menarche rite for herself, at the age of forty-one!

If your first experience of sexual experimentation, masturbation, or intercourse was guilt-ridden or demeaning, rewrite the script. Take who you are and what you know now, then draft a vision of how these events might have taken place in a way that would have been more to

your liking. You may wish to share this with someone special—maybe
your partner or a good friend—so that your revision is witnessed.

Discovering Your Cycle

If you are just now learning about your monthly cycle, certain questions and concerns will probably arise. Most women wonder why no
one ever told them these facts about sex and their bodies before. Do
you feel angry at having been kept in the dark this way? Or do you feel
foolish or inept at never having noticed these cyclic changes in yourself? Or perhaps you simply feel loss and sadness at having missed out
on this aspect of yourself for some period of time? Typically, women
are both disturbed and affirmed to find that romantic feelings attributed to a particular relationship were in large part biological promptings coming from their own bodies at certain times of the month.

You may wish to go back through the questions in the previous
paragraph and examine your feelings more closely, exploring them a
bit in writing. Try to evoke the curious, courageous you, unfettered by
guilt or fear, confidently following your own lead.

Choose this, or another power image of yourself, and bring it to the
task at hand: discovering and trusting your cycle. If you are troubled
with PMS, irregular or painful menses, or infertility that has no
apparent physical cause, ask your wise self for counsel. Do this in
writing, song, meditation, or dreams.

If you feel completely out of touch, can't remember anything, or
are upset by this exercise, refer to Chapter 9, particularly the checklist
on sexual abuse.

If your cycle is basically smooth and trouble-free, take a moment to
consider why. Do you follow any particular menstrual routine or

ritual? Cultural mores view menstrual blood on a spectrum from filthy to sacred. How do you feel about your blood? Do you enjoy and make the most of your fertile time? How so? How do you benefit most from paying attention to your cycle? And what do you have yet to learn and do to more fully honor your rhythms?

If you feel you are fairly complete with this area of investigation, single out any aspects that remain troublesome or unsettled for you. These are your carryover issues. As you move through the next stages, you will be able to view these issues in new contexts, which may help you better cope with them.

Pregnant for the First Time

Having your first baby? Then you have much to contemplate and decide. You may have already discovered that pregnancy is a social event. You are probably being bombarded with questions, advice, or even physical contact (belly touching) from absolute strangers. This, you can't avoid. In fact, if you are able to stay open and objective, you may use these encounters to learn more about your beliefs and conditioning, particularly if you feel yourself being triggered by another's words or actions.

Let's look at your background more closely. What did your mother tell you about birth? How did you react? What about your grandmother or other female relatives? Try to recollect your feelings at these moments of revelation. If you were to summon each of these women now to stand before you, what sort of wisdom might each impart about how to cope with labor?

Control is a major issue in childbearing. How do you feel about losing control? About being and appearing vulnerable? How do you think you might behave if the pain really got to you? What kinds of things could your partner or care provider do to help you feel better? What could you do to help yourself? Do any of these relate to your sensual and sexual likes and dislikes?

Look at the last few questions, and see if there are any ideas you can share with your partner or care provider. For example, maybe you love to have your hair stroked, or your head held, or your feet rubbed, but nobody knows this except you. Pregnancy is the time to make these desires known, absolutely.

Fantasize about yourself in labor. Where are you? Is it dark, light, noisy, or quiet? Who is with you, and what are they doing? What are you doing? What position are you in, how are you breathing, and how do you feel?

Now imagine your labor suddenly getting much stronger. Wow—it really hurts! How do you react? Do you open up, or close down? Do you reach out for help, or withdraw? Relate these responses to your experience of sex. What do you do when it stops feeling good, either emotionally or physically? Women sometimes think they want to have sex even though they feel themselves shutting down. Think about the times this has happened to you. Was it really sex you wanted, or something else? Crack the code on this matter, and you will discover the kind of support you are most likely to need in labor.

How do you handle being sexually frustrated? Do you ask for what you want, get angry, sulk, or just withdraw? Take the opportunity while pregnant to begin asking for what you need, when you need it, in every possible area of your life, and especially in bed. This is core preparation for giving birth.

Finally, how do you respond when others try to tell you what's good for you? Do you clam up and keep the peace, become angry, or assert your position? With regard to extraneous advice during labor, or procedures you do not want, how do you think you might respond? What do you think would be most effective?

Pregnant Again?

◎

Whether carrying your second, third, or fourth baby, you will probably have issues remaining from your other birth experiences that merit attention. Did you feel in any way violated during your birth experience? Were things done to you or the baby without your permission, or that you did not desire? Was your privacy invaded? Did you feel powerless, unsupported, ridiculed, or ridiculous in a way you can't let go of? Were promises broken by your care provider? Do you feel that they abandoned you during or after the birth?

If any of the above fit, you may want to write a letter to the appropriate party or parties. Whether you choose to send it or not, writing it will be therapeutic. I personally think it is critical to let your care provider know how you feel—critical for you, for them, and for all the women they serve.

How was your partner during the whole experience? Did he or she let you down or disappoint you in any way? Do you have feelings about what happened between you during labor that you have never shared? Did the birth affect your sex life or intimacy? Again, a letter is a good place to start; it can help you sort through your thoughts and feelings before you begin to discuss them.

If your partner's behavior during the birth links to some long-term problem that the two of you have been over many times, you may be ripe for counseling. Perhaps you see the need, but can you assert it to your partner? If not, you may be bound by feelings of unworthiness or a lack of self-esteem. Perhaps you have a history of abuse. You need support and an opportunity to express yourself, either one-on-one with a counselor or in group therapy.

Don't wait to begin this work—do it now. Read widely, and educate yourself on your birth options. Communicate your hopes and desires to your partner and care provider, and your next experience could be the birth of your dreams!

Newly Postpartum

◎

If you are newly or recently postpartum, you may be struggling with feelings of dependency. Often these arise during labor, although you may not have recognized them as such. Feelings of dependency are strongly linked to fears of abandonment.

Let us not confuse dependency with vulnerability. Vulnerability is normal in labor; it is actually a desired state. It is characterized by high levels of sensitivity, openness, and receptivity. In contrast, dependency is marked by feelings of not being able to rely on yourself, of needing others to define your reality.

Hospital policies and personnel often engender feelings of dependency in patients so that they will be compliant. Highly invasive or unnecessary procedures exacerbate these feelings. If a woman feels that she has lost her power in labor, she will likely feel abandoned by those who stood by and let it happen. Or she may feel that it was all her fault.

Here are some questions to help you sort out this out. Did you make your best attempt to educate yourself during pregnancy, and to set up your birth situation in advance? Did you inform those on your birth team—your partner, care provider, and other intimates—of your plans and wishes? If so, work through your disappointment as suggested in the previous section, or just let it be—it is certainly not your fault.

Or, did you find it hard to focus on your own needs while pregnant? Did you feel less and less communicative as pregnancy progressed? If things were done during labor that you did not want, did you think it was all your fault? Do you often feel that everyone has power but you? Do you find yourself becoming deeply upset or anxious if people pull away from or reject you? Affirmative answers to these questions link strongly to a history of abuse, or to drug or alcohol dependency. Get help for this.

Regarding the postpartum period, there is yet another category of abuse to consider: that perpetrated by society. In Chapter 5, we looked at the routine abandonment of new mothers in the United States. Even women who have led relatively stable lives may find themselves exhibiting symptoms of anxiety and depression at this juncture.

Generally, the solution is as much a matter of practical assistance with recovery and household responsibilities as of emotional support.

But some women are barely able to tolerate the basic vulnerability of motherhood. Before the birth, did you resolve that your baby would disrupt your life as little as possible? Did you choose to have medication very early in labor? If given your baby immediately at birth, did you experience feelings of ambivalence? Were (or are) you anxious to get back to work at once? Fear of motherhood is often linked to limited amounts of support, love, and affection in the childhood household. What was your mother's attitude toward child rearing? Was she long-suffering, with predominantly negative views of menstruation, childbearing, and sexuality? Do you often feel upset or uncomfortable when caring for your baby? If so, frustration can build to dangerous levels and may even lead to violence. Get help. Make an anonymous call to a women's hotline or counseling referral service as soon as possible.

We have already discussed postpartum sexual frustrations. Are you perhaps compounding these with negative feelings about your body? Do you find your copious secretions (milk, lochia, sweat) offensive? Do you feel ashamed that you look a bit softer and plumper than usual? Or do you take pride in your body for all it has accomplished: birth, breast-feeding, day-by-day recovery, and care of your newborn?

Has your weight been an issue for most of your adult life? If so, you will probably be somewhat unhappy postpartum. Do you have a history of eating disorders? Nothing is worse for you and your baby than dieting while breast-feeding; in fact, you need more calories than you did while pregnant. Exercise is the answer, even though it takes a while to find the time and energy for a workout.

A few other considerations: Do you feel conflict between being a mother and being sexual? Where do you think this comes from? What were your mother's beliefs in this regard? What are your partner's attitudes on the subject? At first, it feels awkward to swing so dramatically from erotic to maternal feelings, but as the baby grows and privacy returns, these feelings settle into their respective places.

The primary question postpartum is this: Can you give yourself permission to change and grow? Do you trust your body to tell you what to eat and drink and when to rest? Do you believe that your body will fully recover in good time? Or do you feel that your body has betrayed you? Have others told you outright that your body is not up to par, not good enough? Think of every individual who has told you this throughout your lifetime, and explore your response to each. Can you let go of your anger and find forgiveness?

Keep a journal of your daily accomplishments at this stage, noting in particular the ways in which your body works for you. Pay special attention to the times you feel physically well and wonderful, and write about them, too.

Juggling Career, Family, and Intimacy

◎

The work to be done in the area of juggling a career, a family, and intimacy can probably be summed up in a single question: What are your priorities? You may be able to learn more about our own values if you examine the priorities of your parents. Are you emulating or reacting to them, or are you truly self-determined?

Ever since the 1950s, women have typically attempted to do too much. How was it in your household? What messages did you get from your mother and father regarding responsibility for the housework? Responsibility for children? Responsibility for emotional issues? Responsibility for individual health and well-being?

What was your mother's attitude regarding her own needs? Did she take private time? What were the things she loved to do—just for herself? Did she set boundaries that you and other family members were aware of and respected?

Generally, women tend to make care of the children their top priority, and that is as it should be. But did your mother have any help? What kind, and how often? Do you think it was enough?

This brings us to the subjects of stress and anger. How did your mother handle these emotions? How do you handle them? How does your approach to stress and anger affect you and your loved ones?

What was your parents' attitude about their intimate relationship? Did they show their romantic feelings for each other? Did they make time for their love, apart from you? How open were your parents about sexual matters? What was the basic attitude or feeling about sex in your household? Were your personal boundaries and need for privacy respected by your family?

Take a look at your current weekly workload. You may benefit from writing down all that you do, then calculating the amount of time spent in each general area: career, housework, family interaction, personal pursuits, and private time with your partner. Play with this on paper, look at any obvious imbalance, then reallocate your time to suit your needs right now. Many of us believe ourselves to be trapped by necessity in unsatisfying expenditures of time, when in fact these are simply a matter of habit. Women at this stage of life must recognize that there will never be enough time to do and have it all. Your priorities can and should change from day to day, week to week, month to month, year to year. Consider developing a one-year plan, five-year plan, and ten-year plan as a means to be more in touch with your intent in life.

If this seems extremely difficult for you, look back at the questions in this chapter that concern your self-esteem. Do you see patterns of putting yourself down, setting your own needs aside? Perhaps if you can determine when and to whom you give up your power, you will be able to figure out why.

Passing Through Menopause

As mentioned in Chapter 7, your responses as you pass through menopause are likely to reflect those of female relatives, particularly your mother. What did she experience at menopause? Is there anything about her experience that you personally remember? Since most women tend to hide their symptoms, you may want to ask her about any erratic behavior you recall and see what the two of you can piece together.

Moving to yet another area: How do you feel about the passing of your youth? Do you see youth as a state of mind, one that can be maintained indefinitely? If so, what are you doing to keep yourself young and vital? How well are you keeping up with your own interests? How about your spiritual life?

How are you caring for your body at this point? Take inventory of all that you do to stay fit and attractive. Truthfully, are any of these practices a waste of time and money? What does seem to work for you, and how can you place greater emphasis on it?

Have you talked to your partner about your fears and anxieties at this stage of life? Has she or he been supportive? As the hormonal surges of menopause move you ever closer to your deepest concerns and longings, do you find that you can share these with your partner? And how do you use your visions? Are you incorporating them into your life, or merely coping?

Think about where you want to go after "the change." Can you use your menopausal energy as a springboard to expand your life? Who are your closest allies in this process? How can you make the most of the support they offer?

Growing Older and Wiser

How do you feel about growing older? What do you still look forward to experiencing or accomplishing? How about your partner? Have you discussed your rounding-out goals and dreams with one another?

What lessons do you have yet to learn in life? Are there challenging situations that keep repeating themselves? What will it take for you to move through them? Can you deliberately set the stage for this, and to what degree are you willing to do so? Who are your best allies for confronting these challenges?

With regard to sex: How is your communication with your partner? Are you happy with yourself sexually? More or less so than before? In terms of sexual self-expression, are there things you would still like to try to do? How do you think your partner would react?

Look closely at yourself now, and look back to where you have been. Are there ways you still don't feel comfortable with your body? Are there parts of your body you never learned to love? Are there sexual wounds or criticisms you have never healed? See whether or not you need to be witnessed, or if you can find a way to embrace yourself fully on your own. In terms of longevity, a healthy body is an integrated body.

How are your relationships with your grown children? Are you comfortable sharing ideas with them, or do you feel misplaced? Identify your Crone aspect: wise, objective, and irrevocably frank. When the Crone speaks, she does so from a point of clarity and certitude. Feel the difference between whining or cajoling and speaking the truth, without expectations.

Do you have many outlets for your accumulated wisdom? Can you find any more? Your vitality is strongly linked to your self-expression.

Have you considered taking the role of family historian? If you have not done so already, you might begin assembling and organizing papers and photographs into albums, adding your own narrative if you like. Each of your children can have his or her own album, and there may also be a composite one that includes the family tree. All of these will be treasured by your offspring, and creating them will give you some closure in certain areas of your life.

In Summary

Now that you have had the opportunity to reflect on each phase of life you've already experienced, and have read about others yet to come, perhaps you have discovered some underlying themes in your sexual story, woven from your family history, ways that culture has affected you, and all you have done on your path of self-discovery. Remember the definition of sexuality given earlier: for a woman, sexuality is all that it means to be female. This is the key to both pleasure and intimacy—bringing all of yourself to your sexual encounters.

Our journey as women through this particular period of history is tremendously rich and complex. Keeping an overview of the cycles and stages in life can help us keep our wits about us, retain a sense of humor, and become wise. And, as men become more concerned with finding balance in their own lives, it has never been more important, or in many ways easier, to articulate all that it means to be a woman.

But we have a long way to go. Far too many women live in poverty, abusive situations, or other conditions of hardship for us to become complacent. We have so much to do, so much to speak and write about, so much to share across the generations. May our sexual vitality and capacity for intimacy infuse these tasks with passion, commitment, and love. And may we readily find courage at every crossroad.

Notes

Author's Note

1. Helen Fisher, *The First Sex: The Natural Talents of Women and How They Are Changing the World* (New York: Ballantine Books, 1999).

2. Ibid.

Chapter 1

1. Nancy Friday, *Women on Top* (New York: Pocket Books, 1991).

2. Natalie Angier, *Woman: An Intimate Geography* (New York: Anchor Books, 1999).

3. Sheila Kitzinger, *Woman's Experience of Sex* (New York: Penguin Putnam Inc., 1985).

4. Hallie Iglehart, *Woman Spirit* (San Francisco: Harper & Row, 1983).

5. Barbara Walker, *The Crone* (San Francisco: Harper & Row, 1985).

6. Susan Griffin, *Pornography and Silence* (New York: Harper & Row, 1981).

7. *Webster's New Collegiate Dictionary*, (1969), s.v "sexuality."

8. Anne Moir and David Jessel, *Brain Sex* (New York: Carol Publishing Group, 1991).

9. Camille Paglia, quoted in "Hurricane Camille Wreaks Havoc," *San Francisco Chronicle*, September, 1992.

10. Moir and Jessel, *Brain Sex.*

11. Christiane Northrup, *Women's Bodies, Women's Wisdom*, rev. ed. (New York: Bantam, 1999).

12. Laura Allen and Roger A. Gorski, "Sexual Dimorphism of the Anterior Commissure and the Massa Intermedia of the Human Brain," *Journal of Comparative Neurology* 312 (1991).

Allen and Gorski, "Sex Differences in the Corpus Callosum of the Living

Human Being," *Journal of Neuroscience* 11:4 (1991).

13. John Gray, *Men, Women and Relationships: Making Peace with the Opposite Sex* (Portland, OR: Beyond Words Publishing, 1990).

Chapter 2

1. Carol Gilligan, *In a Different Voice: Psychological Theory of Women's Development* (Cambridge, MA: Harvard University Press, 1982).

2. Joan Borysenko, audiotape, *"The Woman's Book of Life."*

3. Gilligan, *In a Different Voice: Psychological Theory of Women's Development.*

4. Elizabeth Davis and Carol Leonard, *The Women's Wheel of Life: Thirteen Archetypes of Woman at Her Fullest Power* (New York: Penguin/Putnam, 1996).

5. Theresa L. Crenshaw, *The Alchemy of Love and Lust* (New York: Pocket Books, 1996).

6. Natalie Angier, *Woman: An Intimate Geography* (New York: Anchor Books, 1999).

7. Robin Baker and Mark A. Bellis, *Human Sperm Competition: Copulation, Masturbation and Infidelity* (New York: Chapman & Hall, 1996).

8. Angier, *Woman: An Intimate Geography.*

9. Ibid.

10. David Cohen, *The Circle of Life* (New York: HarperCollins, 1991).

11. Cohen, *The Circle of Life.*

Chapter 3

1. Helen Fisher, *The First Sex* (New York: Ballantine Books, 1999).

2. "Women Score High During Ovulation," *San Francisco Chronicle*, 1985.

3. Winnifred B. Cutler, *Love Cycles* (New York: Villard Books, 1991).

4. Christiane Northrup, *Women's Bodies, Women's Wisdom*, rev. ed. (New York: Bantam Books, 1998).

5. Fisher, *The First Sex*.

6. Joan Borysenko, audiotape, *"The Woman's Book of Life."*

7. Theresa L. Crenshaw, *The Alchemy of Love and Lust* (New York: Pocket Books, 1996).

8. Barbara G. Walker, *The Woman's Encyclopedia of Myths and Secrets* (San Francisco: Harper & Row, 1983).

9. Judy Grahn, *Blood, Bread, and Roses* (Boston: Beacon Press, 1993).

10. Dena Taylor, *Red Flower: Rethinking Menstruation* (Freedom, CA: Crossing Press, 1988).

11. Penelope Shuttle and Peter Redgrove, *The Wise Wound* (New York: Richard Marek, 1978).

12. Dena Taylor, *Red Flower: Rethinking Menstruation.*

13. Crenshaw, *The Alchemy of Love and Lust.*

14. Mary Jane Sherfey, *The Nature and Evolution of Female Sexuality* (New York: Random House, 1973).

15. Walker, *The Woman's Encyclopedia of Myths and Secrets.*

16. Northrup, *Women's Bodies, Women's Wisdom.*

17. C. Wedekind, T. Seeback, F. Bettens, and A. J. Paepke, "MHC-Dependent Mate Preferences in Humans," in *Proceedings of the Royal Society of London* (1995).

18. S. Sumiala et al., "Salivary Progesterone Concentration After Tubal Sterilization," *Obstetrics and Gynecology*, vol. 88 (1996).

19. Luisa Francia, *Dragontime* (New York: Ash Tree Publishing, 1988).

Chapter 4

1. Niles Newton and Charlotte Modahl, "New Frontiers of Oxytocin Research," in *Free Woman: Women's Health in the 1990s*. Eds. E.V. Van Hall and W. Everaerd (Canforth, England: Parthenon Publishing Group, 1989).

2. Ina May Gaskin, *Spiritual Midwifery*, 3d ed. (Summertown, TN: Book Publishing Co., 1990).

3. Niles Newton, Michael Newton, and Donald Foshee, "Experimental Inhibition of Labor Through Environmental Disturbance," *Obstetrics and Gynecology*, vol. 27 (1966).

4. Grantly Dick-Read, *Childbirth Without Fear* (New York: Harper & Row, 1959).

5. Michel Odent, *Water and Sexuality* (London: Penguin Books, 1990).

6. Roberto Caldeyro-Barcia, "The Influence of Maternal Bearing-down Efforts During Second Stage on Fetal Well-being," *Birth and the Family Journal*, vol. 6, no. 1 (spring 1979).

7. Sheila Kitzinger, *Woman's Experience of Sex* (New York: Penguin Putnam Inc., 1985).

8. E. B. Keverne, F. Levy, P. Poindron, and D. R. Lindsay, "Vaginal Stimulation: An Important Determinant of Maternal Bonding in Sheep," *Science*, vol. 219 (1983).

9. D. Krehbiel, P. Poindron, F. Levy, and M. J. Podhomme, "Peridural Anesthesia Disturbs Maternal Behavior in Primiparous and Multiparous Parturient Ewes," *Physiology and Behavior*, vol. 40 (1982).

Chapter 5

1. Niles Newton and Charlotte Modahl, "Mood State Differences Between Breast and Bottle-Feeding Mothers," in *Newton on Breastfeeding* (Seattle: Birth and Life Bookstore, 1990).

2. E. B. Thoman, A. Wetzel, and S. Levine, "Lactation Prevents Disruption of

Temperature Regulation and Suppresses Adrenocortical Activity in Rats," *Communicative Behavior in Biology*, vol. 2, part A (1968).

3. Niles Newton, "The Role of the Oxytocin Reflexes in Three Interpersonal Reproductive Acts: Coitus, Birth and Breastfeeding," in *Newton on Breastfeeding*.

4. Gloria Steinem, *Revolution from Within* (Boston: Little, Brown, 1992).

5. W. H. Masters and V. E. Johnson, *Human Sexual Response* (Boston: Little, Brown, 1966).

6. Kerstin Uvnas-Moberg, "The Role of Efferent and Afferent Vagal Nerve Activity During Reproduction: Integrating Function of Oxytocin on Metabolism and Behavior," *Psychoneuroendocrinology*, vol. 19 (1994).

Chapter 6

1. Camille Paglia, quoted in "Hurricane Camille Wreaks Havoc," *San Francisco Chronicle*, September, 1992.

2. Elizabeth Davis and Carol Leonard, *The Women's Wheel of Life: Thirteen Archetypes of Woman at Her Fullest Power* (New York: Penguin Putnam Inc., 1996).

3. John Gray, *Men, Women and Relationships* (Hillsboro, OR: Beyond Words Publishing, 1990).

4. M. F. Belenky, B. M. Clinchy, N. R. Goldberg, and J. M. Tarule, *Women's Ways of Knowing* (New York: Basic Books, 1986).

5. Marilyn Ruman, "Sex and Anger," *New Woman*, April 1991.

6. Gray, *Men, Women and Relationships*.

7. Davis and Leonard, *The Women's Wheel of Life*.

8. T. Berry Brazelton, *Infants and Mothers* (New York: Delacorte Press, 1969).

9. Pepper Schwartz, *Peer Marriage: How Love Between Equals Really Works* (New York: The Free Press, 1994).

10. Andrew Ward, *Out Here* (New York: Penguin Books, 1991).

11. June Reinisch, "The Kinsey Report" (syndicated), *San Francisco Chronicle*, 1990.

Chapter 7

1. Robert A. Wilson, *Feminine Forever* (New York: Pocket Books, 1971).

2. David Reuben, *Everything You Always Wanted to Know About Sex but Were Afraid to Ask* (New York: Bantam Books, 1971).

3. Sheila Kitzinger, *Woman's Experience of Sex* (New York: Penguin Putnam Inc., 1985).

4. Susan Lark, *The Menopause Self-Help Book* (Berkeley, CA: Celestial Arts, 1992).

5. Joan Borysenko, audiotape, *"The Woman's Book of Life."*

6. Borysenko, Ibid.

7. Borysenko, Ibid.

8. "Menopause: Baby Boomers' Next Step," *The Los Angeles Times*, December 1989.

9. F. Grodstein et al., "Postmenopausal Hormone Therapy and Mortality," *New England Journal of Medicine*, vol. 336, no. 25 (1997).

10. J. Jeppesen et al., "Effects of Low-Fat, High-Carbohydrate Diets on Risk Factors for Ischemic Heart Disease in Postmenopausal Women," *American Journal of Clinical Nutrition*, vol. 65 (1997).

11. Elizabeth Davis and Carol Leonard, *The Women's Wheel of Life: Thirteen Archetypes of Woman at Her Fullest Power* (New York: Penguin Putnam Inc., 1996).

12. Susun Weed, *Menopausal Years: The Wise Woman Way* (Portland, OR: Ash Tree Publishing, 1993).

13. Barbara Raskin, *Hot Flashes* (New York: St. Martin's Press, 1987).

14. Winnifred Culter, *Love Cycles* (New York: Villard Books, 1991).

15. "Why Organic Food Matters," *The Journal of Sustainable Agriculture*, vol. 1, no. 1 (1985).

16. Lois Jovanovic and Genell Subak-Sharpe, *Hormones: The Woman's Answer Book*, (New York: Ballantine, 1987).

17. Christiane Northrup, *Women's Bodies, Women's Wisdom*, rev. ed. (Bantam Books: New York, 1999).

18. Dena Taylor, *Red Flower: Rethinking Menstruation* (Freedom, CA.: Crossing Press, 1988).

19. Barbara Walker, *The Crone* (San Francisco: Harper & Row, 1985).

20. Luisia Francia, *Dragontime* (New York: Ash Tree Publishing, 1988).

21. Zsuzsanna Budapest, *Holy Book of Women's Mysteries* (Berkeley, CA: Wingbow Press, 1989).

22. Barbara Myerhoff, "By Means of Performance," in *Celebration: Studies in Festivity and Ritual*, ed. Victoria Turner (Washington, DC: Smithsonian Institution Press, 1982).

Chapter 8

1. Barbara Walker, *The Crone* (San Francisco: Harper & Row, 1985).

2. Barbara Ehrenreich and Deirdre English, *Witches, Midwives and Nurses: A History of Women Healers* (New York: Feminist Press, 1973).

3. Walker, *The Crone*.

4. Natalie Angier, *Woman: An Intimate Geography* (New York: Anchor Books, 1999).

5. Kristin Hawkes, J. F. O'Connell, and N. G. Burton, "The Grandmother Hypothesis and Human Evolution," in *Adaptation and Evolutionary Biology*,

ed. L. Cronk et al. (New York: Aldine de Gruyter, forthcoming); Kristin Hawkes, J. F. O'Connell, and N. G. Burton, "Hazda Women's Time Allocation, Offspring Provisioning, and the Evolution of Long Postmenopausal Lifespans," *Current Anthropology*, vol. 38 (1997).

6. Luisa Francia, *Dragontime* (New York: Ash Tree Publishing, 1988).

7. Rhonda L. Winn and Niles Newton, "Sexuality in Aging: A Study of 106 Cultures," *Archives of Sexual Behavior*, vol. 2, no. 4 (1982).

8. Jerry Gerber, Janet Wolff, Walter Klores, and Gene Brown, *Life Trends* (New York: Avon Books, 1989).

9. Gerber et al., *Life Trends*.

10. Gerber et. al., *Life Trends*.

11. Sheila Kitzinger, *Woman's Experience of Sex* (New York: Penguin Putnam, Inc., 1985).

Chapter 9

1. Laura Davis and Ellen Bass, *The Courage to Heal* (New York: Harper & Row, 1988).

2. Sheila Kitzinger, *Woman's Experience of Sex* (New York: Penguin Books, 1985).

3. Christiane Northrup, *Women's Bodies, Women's Wisdom*, rev. ed. (New York: Bantam Books, 1999).

4. Beverly Engel, *The Emotionally Abused Woman* (Los Angeles: Lowell House, 1990).

5. Avodah K. Offit, *The Sexual Self* (New York: J. B. Lippincott, 1977).

6. Engel, *The Emotionally Abused Woman*.

7. Offit, *The Sexual Self*.

8. Robin Baker and Mark A. Bellis, *Human Sperm Competition: Copulation,*

Masturbation and Infidelity (New York: Chapman & Hall, 1996).

9. Helen Fisher, *The First Sex: The Natural Talents of Women and How They Are Changing the World* (New York: Ballantine Books, 1999).

10. Barbara Walker, *The Women's Encyclopedia of Myths and Secrets* (New York: Harper & Row, 1988).

Chapter 10

1. Phyllis Chesler, *Women and Madness* (New York: Avon Books, 1973).

2. Winnifred Cutler, *Love Cycles* (New York: Villard Books, 1991).

3. Anne Moir and David Jessel, *Brain Sex* (New York: Carol Publishing, 1991).

Index

THE FERTILITY AWARENESS HANDBOOK: The Natural Guide to Avoiding or Achieving Pregnancy
by Barbara Kass-Annese, R.N., C.N.P., and Hal Danzer, M.D.

Do you know your fertility signs? Do you know that they can help you to track the days of the month when you are most fertile and likely to conceive or are infertile and can safely have intercourse without conceiving?

This richly illustrated book gives step-by-step instructions for using fertility awareness methods, from taking your basal temperature to charting ovulation. These non-invasive techniques have no side effects and teach you how to be more in touch with your body and in control of your health and sexual well-being.

160 pages ... 47 illus. ... Paperback $11.95 ... 5th Edition

GETTING PREGNANT AND STAYING PREGNANT: Overcoming Infertility and Managing Your High-Risk Pregnancy *by* Diana Raab, B.S., R.N. Revised 3rd Edition

This is a practical guide to the physical, medical, and emotional issues women and their partners face during infertility treatments and high-risk pregnancies. Winner of the 1992 Benjamin Franklin Award for Best Health Book, this book combines accurate medical information with a nurse's thoughtfulness and care. It covers new infertility technologies, tests, and genetic risks, and combines information about what to expect during a high-risk pregnancy with supportive ideas for coping with cesareans, miscarriages, and premature births.

320 pages ... 11 illus. ... Paperback ... $15.95

THE A-TO-Z OF PREGNANCY AND CHILDBIRTH
by Nancy Evans

This book will answer all your questions about medical and other issues surrounding pregnancy and childbirth. It offers clear discussions of topics such as infertility treatments and reproductive technology, breastfeeding and its effects on mother and baby, and home vs. hospital birth. The alphabetical entries are supplemented with numerous illustrations, charts, and practical tips. A special *two-color foldout chart shows monthly fetal and maternal development at each month of pregnancy*.

352 pages ... 21 illus. ... Paperback ... $16.95 ... Hard cover $29.95

To order or for our FREE catalog call (800) 266-5592

ONCE A MONTH: Understanding and Treating PMS
by Katharina Dalton, M.D. Revised 6th Edition

Once considered an imaginary complaint, PMS has at last received the serious attention it deserves, thanks largely to the work of Katherine Dalton, M.D. One-third of the material is new in this sixth edition, from the latest research on how PMS affects learning to the PMS-menopause connection. Most importantly, Dr. Dalton addresses the whole range of possible treatments—from self-care methods such as the three-hourly starch diet and relaxation techniques to the newest medical options, including updated guidelines for progesterone therapy.

320 pages ... 55 illus. ... Paperback $15.95

ANDROGEN DISORDERS IN WOMEN: The Most Neglected Hormone Problem *by* Theresa Cheung

One in ten women in the U.S. suffers from an imbalance of the so-called "male hormones" known as androgens. Effects include excessive facial or body hair, unusual hair loss, severe acne, dull skin, fatigue, weight gain, menstrual dysfunction, ovarian cysts, and infertility. Because women are often embarassed by the effects and doctors tend to dismiss or ignore the symptoms, there has been little discussion about androgen disorders—until now. This book describes the medical and emotional effects that excessive androgens can have and outlines the various forms of conventional and alternative treatment.

224 pages ... Paperback $13.95 ... Hard cover $23.95

MENOPAUSE WITHOUT MEDICINE
by Linda Ojeda, Ph.D. ... New 4th Edition

Linda Ojeda broke new ground 15 years ago with this bestselling resource on menopause, giving women a clear understanding of menopausal changes and guidelines for effective self-care.

In this new edition, she re-examines the hormone therapy debate; suggests natural remedies for depression, hot flashes, sexual changes, and skin and hair problems; and presents an illustrated basic exercise program. She also includes up-to-date information on natural sources of estrogen, including phytoestrogens, and how diet and personality affect mood swings.

352 pages ... 32 illus. ... 62 tables ... Paperback $15.95... Hard cover $25.95

All prices subject to change

SENSUAL SEX: Awakening Your Senses and Deepening the Passion in Your Relationship
by Beverly Engel, MFCC

Life is a sensual experience that asks us to stop and listen, smell, taste, touch—and enjoy. *Sensual Sex* is about slow, sensuous, artful loving that feels good to both partners. The one-of-a-kind "Reawakening Your Senses" program engages couples in a whole new level of physical exploration, "Deeper Love" offers an introduction to Tantric sex and sexual ecstasy; and "The Four Seasons of Sensuous Passion" discusses the stages of a long-term intimate relationship and sensual exercises that can strengthen each phase. Sensitively written and beautifully designed, this is a book to share, enjoy, and keep for a long time.

256 pp. ... Paperback $14.95

SEXUAL PLEASURE: Reaching New Heights of Sexual Arousal and Intimacy *by* Barbara Keesling, Ph.D.

Sexual Pleasure takes the reader through a series of stimulating exercises, done alone and with a partner, to increase sensual awareness and experience sexual intimacy. These exercises can be used by people of any sexual orientation and by those who may have physical limitations or are just learning about their sexuality—anyone seeking the secrets of strong and fulfilling sex.

"For anyone who wishes to increase the ability to experience sensual pleasure." — Yoga Journal

224 pp. ... 14 b/w photos ... Paperback $13.95 ... Hard cover $21.95

MAKING LOVE BETTER THAN EVER: Reaching New Heights of Passion and Pleasure After 40
by Barbara Keesling, Ph.D.

In this book, Dr. Barbara Keesling shows couples how to reignite sexual feelings while reconnecting emotionally. She provides a series of relaxation, body-image, and caress exercises that demonstrate the power of touch to heighten sexual response and expand sexual potential; reduce anxiety and increase health and well-being; build self-esteem and improve body image; open the lines of communication; and promote playfulness, spontaneity, and a natural sense of joy.

208 pp. ... 14 b/w photos ... Paperback $13.95 ... Hard cover $24.95

To order see last page or call (800) 266-5592

ORDER FORM

10% DISCOUNT on orders of $50 or more —
20% DISCOUNT on orders of $150 or more —
30% DISCOUNT on orders of $500 or more —
On cost of books for fully prepaid orders

NAME

ADDRESS

CITY/STATE   ZIP/POSTCODE

PHONE   COUNTRY (outside of U.S.)

TITLE	QTY	PRICE	TOTAL
Women's Sexual Passages (paperback)		@ $15.95	

Prices subject to change without notice

Please list other titles below:

		@ $	
		@ $	
		@ $	
		@ $	
		@ $	
		@ $	
		@ $	
		@ $	

Check here to receive our book catalog   ❏   free

Shipping Costs

First book: $3.00 by bookpost, $4.50 by UPS, Priority Mail, or to ship outside the U.S.
Each additional book: $1.00
For rush orders and bulk shipments call us at (800) 266-5592

TOTAL	_____
Less discount @____%	(_____)
TOTAL COST OF BOOKS	_____
CA residents add 7½% sales tax	_____
Shipping & handling	_____
TOTAL ENCLOSED	_____

Please pay in U.S. funds only

❏ Check ❏ Money Order ❏ Visa ❏ MasterCard ❏ Discover

Card #_____ Exp. date_____

Signature_____

Complete and mail to:
Hunter House Inc., Publishers
PO Box 2914, Alameda CA 94501-0914
Website: www.hunterhouse.com
Orders: (800) 266-5592 or email: ordering@hunterhouse.com
Phone (510) 865-5282 Fax (510) 865-4295

WSP 12/2000